SUPER
BODY

The information in this book is not intended to constitute medical advice, nor is it intended to replace or conflict with the advice given to you by your doctor or other health professional. Before embarking on the plans set out in this book you should discuss them with your doctor, especially if you have any medical condition or if you are taking any medication. The authors and publisher disclaim any liability directly or indirectly from the use of the material in this book by any person.

SUPER BODY

A THREE-WEEK PROGRAM
TO HARNESS THE
NEW SCIENCE OF
BODY COMPOSITION
AND RESTORE YOUR
YOUTHFUL CONTOURS

DR WILLIAM DAVIS

yellow
kite

First published in Great Britain in 2025 by Yellow Kite
An imprint of Hodder & Stoughton Limited
An Hachette UK company

SRD

Cover design by Jim Datz
Cover image by Shutterstock
Cover copyright © 2025 by Hachette Book Group, Inc.
Images on pages 12, 14 and 15 from Shutterstock

A CIP catalogue record for this title is available from the British Library

Trade Paperback ISBN 978 1 399 74050 0
ebook ISBN 978 1 399 74051 7

Typeset in Janson Text LT Std

Printed and bound in India by Manipal Technologies Limited, Manipal

Hodder & Stoughton policy is to use papers that are natural, renewable
and recyclable products and made from wood grown in sustainable forests.
The logging and manufacturing processes are expected to conform
to the environmental regulations of the country of origin.

Hodder & Stoughton Limited
Carmelite House
50 Victoria Embankment
London EC4Y 0DZ

www.yellowkitebooks.co.uk

MIX
Paper | Supporting
responsible forestry
FSC™ C104740

CONTENTS

INTRODUCTION

MANY OF US HAVE STRUGGLED WITH VARIOUS DISTORTIONS of body shape. Flabby arms, thick thighs, love handles, double chins, abdominal fat overflowing the sides of an airline seat, Spanx forcing you to play an unpleasant game of Whack-a-Mole, compressing one protuberance only to have another reappear elsewhere—it's not body shaming, but a full-frontal confrontation with what, as a society, so many of us have experienced. Who hasn't struggled with some form of unwanted shape or protuberance of their body? For far too many people, struggling with some aspect of body shape has become the norm, a battle that many have lost. Doctors will often proclaim that our body struggles are genetic. Or they tell us to "move more and eat less." Dietitians advise us to "push the plate away" or "eat many small meals every two hours throughout the day." The media, celebrity culture and influencers, the diet industry, and the dwindling numbers of slender people blame us for lack of willpower, gluttony, and excess. But none of this is true—we are the victims of bad information, misinterpretation, flawed advice.

The pharmaceutical industry tempts us with quick fixes that we inject to eliminate hunger, not informing us that we are either stuck with relying on the drug for a lifetime at considerable health and financial cost, or if we stop the drug, regaining the weight and experiencing a dramatic deterioration in health in its aftermath. The weight regain that inevitably occurs leaves us at *increased* risk for type 2 diabetes and other common health conditions. In *SUPER Body*, I will discuss how and why weight regain is virtually *guaranteed* after stopping the drug, because much of the weight initially lost is muscle, a phenomenon that we now know, given the latest science, ensures that fat will return, *even if a strict reduced-calorie lifestyle and exercise program have been maintained.* The same applies to weight loss achieved by the misery of reducing calories or even a bariatric procedure: Fat weight is regained because much of the weight lost is muscle. Yes—most conventional efforts at weight loss fail to address the critical issue of muscle, ensuring weight regain as fat and thereby leaving us less healthy than we were at the start.

I want to be clear: This is not a book that just criticizes body shape. My goal is to help you understand how and why your body has taken on the shape and composition that it has, and if you are dissatisfied with it, what you can do about it—easily, readily, rapidly, naturally, and inexpensively. As the book title suggests, I will be providing a virtual blueprint that will help you regain lost muscle and lose fat where you don't want it. This method requires no calorie or "point" counting that leaves you desperately hungry, no pharmaceuticals that cause nausea to discourage eating, no bariatric procedures that create peculiar anatomic distortions. It doesn't require plastic surgeons to liposuction off gallons of excess thigh and buttock fat, or ultrasound-shrink double or triple chins. It won't involve smartphone apps that alert you to moments of weakness, to chastise you for encountering eating triggers. It will, however, rely on restoring factors that should have been part of your life all along until modern disruptions—think: antibiotics, food additives, pharmaceuticals, and dietary guidelines—messed up the entire situation, leaving you wondering what the heck happened and at a loss for finding better solutions. We are going to circumvent all the problems that accompany conventional methods of losing weight that do not address the inevitable muscle loss that occurs and shortens your life—yes: shortens your life.

It wasn't that long ago that people would agonize over an issue of appearance that they had little or no control over: the too-large nose inherited from paternal relatives, wide feet for which they struggled to find E-width shoes, intractably curly hair passed down from their mother's Irish side. Those quaint concerns have been replaced by an entirely new collection of struggles, none passed down via genetics, all occurring with epidemic frequency and involving distortions of body form.

Surely, people watchers out there recognized long ago that humans come in a variety of shapes and sizes—shapes and sizes that have undergone a peculiar transformation. It's a phenomenon largely unique to the past half century. There were no XXXL-size dresses and shirts in 1960. Belts usually didn't need to accommodate waists 36 inches or more in circumference. Only two generations ago, 30 pounds of excess weight meant that you were the heaviest among your friends, neighbors, and coworkers. Now, it's more like 100 pounds, even 200 pounds or more. You see it around you: people unable to bend over to tie their shoes, struggling to climb a single flight of stairs, navigating grocery aisles in a motorized shopping cart.

The Centers for Disease Control and Prevention (CDC) tracks these trends, and in 2021, the latest year for which the CDC has tabulated data (as of this writing), 42 percent of Americans fell into the obese range by body mass index (BMI), a measure that divides weight by height, with a BMI of 30 or greater designated "obese." As the obesity situation worsens, doctors have had to come up with new designations such as "super-obese" for people with BMIs of 40 but haven't yet created terms to describe the growing numbers of people with BMIs of 50, 60, or greater. Like a garbage dump that is running out of places to put the flood of incoming trash, the body of a modern human is running out of body locations to store the excess fat, developing odd, never-before-seen protuberances and fat depositions in the heart, knees, hips, pancreas, kidneys, muscle, and elsewhere, locations designated "ectopic fat," a phenomenon that accelerates deterioration of those organs. Doctors come to your rescue by dispensing pharmaceuticals and medical procedures, but never addressing root causes, or by providing dietary advice that ensures your failure. Imagine you start with a BMI of 51 as a 350-pound, 5-foot 9-inch male, undergo a bariatric procedure, and lose an impressive 75 pounds. But, at your new weight of 275 pounds, your BMI is 40—still in the "super-obese" range. Conventional "solutions" to weight loss are not solutions. Like many of the other trappings of modern health care and pharmaceuticals, they are only temporary and incomplete fixes for a much larger problem, problems that, in reality, are easy to address if we abandon the standard approach of a drug or procedure for every health condition.

As a society, have we succumbed to laziness, sloth, and excess, sprouting protuberant body parts that leave us embarrassed, afraid to wear a bathing suit, falling victim to health conditions driven by the fat content of these bulging body parts? Is the modern human body-distorting experience due to weakness and temptation—or is something else at work here in what we consume in the form of antibiotics, food additives, microplastics, PFAS "forever" chemicals, toxic seed oils, sugar-laden sodas, and ultraprocessed food? We didn't just evolve into this state over the last fifty or sixty years.

The bedlam and chaos that define current conventional weight management methods remind me of the way "madness" was managed in the nineteenth century with asylums, straitjackets, bloodletting, and hysterectomies to treat female "hysteria." Such Victorian-age "treatments" were ineffective, of course, barbaric, and inhumane yet were inflicted on countless numbers of people. Modern medical management of weight and body shape is not that far distant from such lamentable historical practices for mental health, practices that hold us hostage with ineffective or, at best, temporarily effective ways to lose weight. No, we should not restrain people with mental illness in straitjackets, nor should we subscribe to conventional approaches to weight loss that ignore the newest science and actually worsen health and appearance.

And it's not just an issue of aesthetics. It is also an issue for emotional health and well-being. Many people who struggle with weight, shape, and body composition view themselves as personal failures. Experiencing the body distortions of modern life can seriously affect self-esteem, faith in your ability to navigate life's problems or attract or maintain a life partner, and even impact your employability. I have had many patients over the years who would emotionally crumble in front of me while sharing their frustrations and disappointments over their perceived inability to lose excess weight or return to something close to a normal body shape. I am haunted, for instance, of memories of a forty-four-year-old woman who, unable to gain control over her emotional eating, resorted to gastric bypass. Two years after her procedure, I sat across from her twenty-two-year-old son, who was sobbing because he found his mom dead in her kitchen from a procedure that, they were assured, was entirely safe and would yield magnificent slenderness with no more than minor risks from the surgery.

You likely did not know that, in the game of weight loss, the odds are fixed against you. Not only did health authorities fail to reveal the real rules to you, they gave you "rules" that should have been discarded as ineffective long ago. You enter the casino with a thousand dollars, blow it all on slots, then leave broke, losing your money to the house since the odds have been stacked against you all along. The odds are even worse in the game of weight loss. By following conventional weight-loss rules, you can enjoy some up-front wins that suck you in, only to experience demoralizing long-term defeats, defeats that leave you not only stuck with regaining the weight you originally lost but with distortions of shape and body composition that impair self-image and health.

It doesn't have to be this way. To win at this game, you need to understand the *real* rules. We begin this path by examining why all the advice given to you by health-care professionals is not just ineffective but *ensures your failure*. You may have paid a lot of money, invested a lot of time and effort, and involved your family in this dietary charade, confident in the wisdom of the doctor or dietitian, only to watch the weight return or find yourself with deteriorating health.

Let's therefore consider the factors absent or lacking in modern life that allow us to acquire distortions of body shape and proportions, causing the shape and body composition of the last two generations to differ dramatically from that of all preceding generations. Thankfully, these are all factors that we are able to restore to ourselves.

Many readers know me from my *Wheat Belly* series of books that discuss the idea that the low-fat era promoting consumption of "healthy whole grains" was a blunder of worldwide proportions, especially since what is now labeled "wheat" is something completely different from the stuff that your grandmother knew. Wheat is now an 18-inch-tall, thick-stalked, large-seeded creation of genetics research. It looks different, is biochemically different, and generates new and unusual effects on unsuspecting humans who consume it. Although created with noble intentions to increase yield per acre for farmers to feed starving worldwide populations, it inadvertently became a monster with altered biochemistry and dangerous health consequences.

Some may also know me from my recent book *Super Gut*, which explains how important microbes have been lost from our microbiome, compromising the very foundation of our health, including how and where fat and muscle are deposited. You may have been labeled with such conditions as depression, anxiety, irritable bowel syndrome, fibromyalgia, or oxalate kidney stones, but much of it is due to disruption of the ecosystem you house in the 30 feet of digestive tract beneath your diaphragm.

SUPER Body is not a repeat of *Wheat Belly* or *Super Gut* ideas. But we all learned so much about weight, appetite, body composition, the microbiome, and overall health from these experiences that it is worth reiterating at least some of these lessons. Insights into body composition have taken some giant steps forward over the decade or so since I upset the dietary world with the *Wheat Belly* arguments. My scientific team and I conducted human clinical trials that yielded dramatic and unexpected findings, pointing to strategies that further modify body shape and composition. I predict that you will be gobsmacked by these insights, many of which you may have never heard before and that have the potential to completely alter your body shape and health. I don't think that it is a stretch to predict that you might look terrific in a bikini at age sixty-five or earn the admiration of onlookers because of your rapid, confident gait that allows you to take the stairs two at a time at age seventy while peers rely on canes, walkers, wheelchairs, or simply succumb to the ravages of aging experienced conventionally, all under the supervision of their doctor.

Conventional methods to achieve weight loss are plagued by the fundamental and crippling problem that people who initially lose weight *regain most or all of the weight lost* over time. This occurs over weeks, months, or even several years—but it inevitably comes back. Weight regain is a phenomenon accompanied by increased risk for serious long-term health consequences, as well as disappointment, disillusionment, and despair. This phenomenon occurs because weight loss achieved by conventional methods involves loss of muscle mass that virtually ensures you have lost control over metabolic rate (i.e., the rate at which you "burn" calories") that will be significantly reduced for many years—not weeks or months, but years. And weight regain is almost entirely fat. If you lose weight accompanied by muscle loss, then regain weight, you have more fat and less muscle than when you started and your risk for health complications, such as heart disease and dementia, are even greater. None of these efforts even begins to address underlying causes so, no surprise, all the weight and the health problems that accompany them come back in full force. If you don't want to follow in the footsteps of your dad or grandfather who had a heart attack followed by bypass surgery, or your mom or grandmother who developed cognitive decline and dementia, eventually not even recognizing their own children—good luck with undoing those processes with conventional efforts at weight loss.

The answers, in reality, are right beneath our noses. Take, for instance, graduates of the television show *The Biggest Loser*. Deprived of calories and encouraged to engage in many hours of aerobic and resistance exercise every day, participants lost extravagant amounts of weight, and by the end of the season, they looked great. But the story doesn't end the way you may think. The majority of successful participants graduated from the show and maintained a reduced-calorie lifestyle and moderate exercise on their return home, only to eventually regain all the weight. After leaving the show, these participants were studied and tracked by a research team from the National Institutes of Health (NIH). The NIH researchers discovered that the show's participants had experienced a profound change in physiology, persisting for years, which virtually guaranteed regain of the weight. Successful, hard-earned weight loss ensured that substantial amounts of fat would return along with feelings of disappointment and defeat, as well as deterioration in measures associated with type 2 diabetes, heart disease, and dementia. You and I can learn from such experiences.

Let's therefore abandon the overly simplistic notion of "losing weight" and, in its place, adopt the notion of improving *body composition*—losing fat from the most important places first; maintaining or even increasing muscle (youthful muscle that you've lost with aging along with muscle lost due to bad weight-loss advice), all without prolonged routines at the gym—and allowing your body to resume its normal business: obtaining optimal body shape, composition, physiology, and health. In that world, there are no "love handles," double chins, XXXL blue jeans, diabetes, hypertension, heart attack, colon cancer, dementia, or snickers over your moral weakness.

In *SUPER Body*, I hope to show readers how restoring a number of factors that we have all lost has potential to undo this untidy mess, no drugs or procedures required. While some of these lessons emerged from the worldwide *Wheat Belly* and *Super Gut* experiences, others originate with new and unexpected observations, including those from my own clinical trials, as well as the growing body of scientific observations coming from other research efforts, all showing us that preservation or increase in muscle is the pivotal difference that prevents weight regain and improves shape and body composition in long-lasting ways. To make it stick, I will share with you a straightforward three-week plan to put these ideas to work to shrink that bulging abdomen, lose the extra chins, bring thighs and buttocks back toward normal contours, and have you shopping in the petite or slim-fit dress or 32-inch-waist pants section again—healthy, vigorous, ambulating on your own without assistance, able to dance the tango or salsa in your most provocative outfit—all without spending excessive hours at the gym.

PART I

PEOPLE OF ALL SHAPES AND SIZES

B UMPY, LUMPY, AND DOWNRIGHT DUMPY." SO THOUGHTLESSLY quipped fashion critic Richard Blackwell about Oprah Winfrey, poking fun at her publicly displayed efforts at managing weight, suffering the ups and downs of trying to re-achieve something closer to an ideal shape. We ought to give her credit for airing her struggles so publicly, even taking a major financial stake in Weight Watchers and serving as a member of their board but, from a shape and body composition perspective, it was all for naught.

But if Oprah, with her vast resources, financial and otherwise, cannot get it right, what hope do you have? If millions of dollars, access to the best personal trainers and nutritionists, and open doors to membership in any gym or weight-loss program still yielded failure after humiliating failure, how can we possibly do any better? Of course, Oprah is not to blame, any more than are all the other millions of people struggling with their bumps and lumps despite following the advice of their doctors and dietitians. They, like Oprah, may also suffer the tactless comments of those gloating over failure. It's yet another example of "Repeat a lie often enough and it becomes the truth"—it was true in Nazi Germany, it's true in our present age of misinformation and disinformation, and it's true in all the popular ideas on how to achieve weight loss. Make no mistake: A lot of money is made delivering the wrong message, over and over again. Whether we label it "semaglutide" or "gastric bypass," these weight-loss methods are all guilty of propagating the same flawed message.

The truth is that you can do far better. But it will involve none of the strategies, tools, or programs that Oprah and millions of others engage in. The menu of strategies that we are going to consider in *SUPER Body* are entirely different, drawing lessons from unexpected places. And our goal is not weight loss per se, but achieving a more desirable redistribution of fat and muscle: shape and body composition, with restoration of youthful musculature, flat abdomens, smoother facial skin—yes: better body contours, but also turning back the clock on agility, vigor, sexual health, and appearance.

In this first section, let's begin by deconstructing all the mistakes made—that continue to be made—by conventional notions of losing weight. We need to dispel deeply held misconceptions so that you are freed from the crippling tyranny of all that you've been told by media, doctors, weight-loss programs, and all the others who continue to propagate messages that, time and again, result in failure.

1

HOW WE GOT SO OUT OF SHAPE

Let's pretend for a moment that we can travel back in time to the year 50,000 BC, some two thousand human generations ago, tens of thousands of years before the appearance of the first human civilizations and cities. Without merchants or shops, without indoor plumbing, without occupational specialization, everyone is a hunter-gatherer, struggling to survive in wild settings, tropical to arctic. Most days, you don your best loincloth and wrap animal skins around your feet to protect them from rocks and twigs, running several miles to hunt, spear, or club prey for your next meal. After all, you and the members of your clan have had nothing to eat except for a few birds' eggs, mushrooms, leaves, and berries the last few days. It's now time to kill something.

You set out, looking for the tracks of animals you recognize as those you can overtake or capture in a trap you planted. You leave at dawn, only to return at sunset, prized kill dragged behind you. You, your family, and clan butcher the creature, hungrily eating some raw, setting aside the rest to roast over a fire. You share the heart, brain, lungs, stomach, intestines, liver, kidneys, meat, skin—yes, everything down to the ligamentous, cartilaginous, bony carcass that remains, heated in water over a fire, adding roots and leaves that other clan members have gathered to make soups or stews, rich in fat and tissue fragments. In

5

this world in which you and your fellow humans work hard to find food, you discard nothing.

Not many people in recent history have had a day like this. Yet this lifestyle of consuming animal body parts provided nutrients that you, living your modern smartphone-enabled, supermarket lifestyle, lack. You don't consume brain or skin, and thereby obtain no hyaluronic acid. You likely don't boil a carcass to mobilize the collagen from cartilage, tendons, and ligaments. Anyone who avoids animal products therefore obtains zero quantities of these body-shaping nutrients as they are exclusively sourced from animal organs, meats, and other body parts. As we shall discuss, increasing your intake of these two factors not only reduces abdominal fat and increases lean muscle mass but also provides significant benefits for the skin, joints, arteries, and brain. Likewise, the modern reliance on fast food, ultraprocessed products, and meaningless dietary guidelines means that dietary intake of body-shaping carotenoids is woefully lacking. Even worse, you've taken multiple courses of antibiotics over the years, and you drink chlorinated water and consume processed foods containing long lists of synthetic additives that have killed or reduced numerous bacterial species in your gastrointestinal microbiome, microbes that played major roles in your shape and body composition.

MOST LIKELY TO SUCCEED: CLASS OF 50,000 BC

For as long as our species, *Homo sapiens*, has walked this planet, we have been fascinated with variations in human body shape. After all, the human body can be a beautiful thing, an engineering marvel capable of spectacular feats: running for hours to track and exhaust an animal during a hunt for food and clothing; using our unique hand construction to fashion tools or create art; having lips, tongue, and vocal cords capable of articulating a wide variety of sounds that we interpret as language or song. We are also uniquely vulnerable without claws or talons, with small incisor teeth ineffective at tearing the neck of prey, nearly hairless, and without hooves; we thereby have to resort to skin and fur scavenged from animals to cover our torsos and feet.

Beneath modern manufactured clothing and shoes we wear, without the incredible communication device we carry in our pocket or purse, and without the societal checks and balances we have that keep our world in working order, more or less, we are really little different from the loincloth-clad, ax-bearing, bloodthirsty *Homo sapiens* of, say, fifty thousand years ago. If we were to compare the genetics of an individual from that era to someone from our own time, there would be no more than a handful of differences. You would be nearly identical, genetically speaking. You may smell better, you may sleep in a nicer bed, and you have ready access to numerous sources of transportation, but, beneath the surface, you are still a wild member of our species. Your basic survival needs are no different, your physiology is the same, your genetic code greater than 99 percent indistinguishable.

But if we were to hold up photos of the class of 50,000 BC against the class of 2000 or thereabouts, we would see stark differences: Humans have experienced dramatic alterations in shape and body composition. We no longer see sinew, six-pack abdominal muscles, or a chiseled neck and chest. In the more recent class photo, we see soft, protuberant, fleshy contours; detail concealed deep under subcutaneous fat; some abdomens so large that they mimic term pregnancy. Probe deeper into our modern class's physical construction and we'll find fat in the liver, fat encircling the small and large intestines, fat in the kidneys, fat surrounding the heart, fat infiltrating joints and muscles—all places where fat does not belong. And there would be many pounds less muscle than our ancient ancestors had, since we don't have to wield weapons to hunt or exert the considerable effort required to skin and gut prey.

But just how relevant is all this to modern life if you don't plan to chase down a gazelle or remove a heart, tongue, and stomach from a wildebeest?

Let's conduct a further thought experiment to illustrate. Imagine that we had a time machine that could retrieve an average human from that era of fifty-thousand-plus years ago. After the initial shock of transporting this poor creature to our world, we open our refrigerators and cupboards to him, treat him to some barbecued ribs and french fries, wake him with the smell of pancakes, let him watch hour after hour of television filled with images of pizza delivered to your doorstep and bowls heaped high with corn chips. He no longer has to sharpen spearheads but can, with a few taps on a phone, order a bucket of fried chicken delivered within minutes to the front door. Who knows what manner of parasites and bacteria this wild-living human carries? After some soap and shampoo, let's treat him with a cocktail of antibiotics and other pharmaceuticals to "clean" him up. It doesn't take long to turn him into a twenty-first-century man: He gains 30 or 40 pounds over a few weeks, his abdomen expands along with bigger thighs, and he develops other fat deposits in his face, neck, chest, pancreas, joints, and elsewhere. Muscles atrophy, sinew no longer visible, facial definition lost, he sighs heavily upon rising from a chair or walking to the refrigerator. No, this graduate of the Paleolithic, preagricultural, precommercial age is no different and every bit as susceptible to all the distortions that modern people have experienced.

Are there lessons to be learned here? I believe there are. Just as a shark or goat or wolf has a specific style of eating programmed into its genetic code that, if violated, leads to rapid deterioration and death, so it goes with *Homo sapiens*. A specific way of living and eating is programmed into our forty-six chromosomes that, as modern people, we have fatally violated. We are paying the price in body shape and composition with peculiar bulges, protuberances, and infiltrations but also an explosion of health conditions, such as type 2 diabetes, heart disease, fatty liver, and colon cancer. It is, yes, about appearance and aesthetics, but it is also about health and disease, mobility, even premature death.

How long would our member of the class of 50,000 BC have lived during his time? Because he survived the high-risk first decade of life, it would be common for him to live to fifty, sixty, or seventy or more years of age without having to experience (what the anthropology community calls) the "diseases of civilization," as we do.[1,2] In his own era, he may have acquired scars from injuries or survived various worm infestations, but his flat abdomen, thickly muscled arms and legs, and ability to climb hills and trees regardless of age permitted none of the many health conditions that have become commonplace in our world. And he did so without counting calories, without benefit of pharmaceuticals or medical procedures, but by adhering to the lifestyle programmed into his genetic code, just like the other wild creatures around him.

NOT ALL FAT IS CREATED EQUAL

There's no Declaration of Independence for fat and, unlike people, all fat is therefore not created equal.

Efforts have been made over the years to decipher just how various deposits of body fat have different health implications. You've likely heard it argued that there are "pear-shaped" and "apple-shaped" people, the former referring to a bottom-heavy body shape with excess fat concentrated mostly in the buttocks and thighs; the latter, to fat accumulating in the abdomen. Being pear-shaped has also been labeled as "gynoid," since premenopausal females are more likely to develop this distribution, whereas being apple-shaped has been labeled "android," as men are more likely to accumulate abdominal fat. After menopause, however, females drift more toward an apple (android) shape due to reduced levels of estrogen. These designations are generalizations, of course, not absolutes, and there can be significant individual variation. In reality, most people are some combination of body types, not a "pure" apple or pear.

Does all this talk of fruit and sex really mean anything? And what consequences does this all have for health? And does it matter?

Conventional methods to characterize shape and body composition have serious flaws. Perhaps your doctor tells you that your body mass index (BMI) is 30, at the start of the obese range, a value obtained by dividing height by weight. But BMI tells you nothing about where the fat is—is it benign fat or is it metabolically dangerous fat? Is it just an aesthetic issue, or are you on track for being diagnosed with type 2 diabetes, a heart attack, or dementia? BMI cannot make that distinction. Athletes or other heavily muscled people will also tell you that, because BMI does not distinguish muscle from fat, tracking BMI is a useless exercise, a misleading gauge of body composition that can label muscular people as overweight or obese. Likewise, consider waist circumference: Is the fat just beneath the skin "subcutaneous" fat, or is it deep within surrounding abdominal organs, "visceral" fat? Waist circumference just tells you that you have fat in the abdominal region, but not exactly where.

It's only over the past couple of decades that these crude distinctions have been deciphered. The turning point in gaining an understanding was largely due to a novel application of cross-sectional computed tomography (CT) and magnetic resonance imaging (MRI), for imaging of the abdomen. These methods clearly delineate the locations of fat, unlike previous body shape–characterizing methods.

There are therefore two main locations, or "compartments," of fat: subcutaneous and abdominal visceral—as different as night and day. Subcutaneous fat is that which collects in the buttocks, thighs, neck, chest, and elsewhere, just beneath the skin. It's the fat that feels spongy when you press on it with a finger. While you may not like the various bulges and protuberances that result from accumulations of subcutaneous fat, this form is only responsible for unpleasant aesthetics and for adding to stress on weight-bearing joints, such as hips and knees.

Abdominal visceral fat surrounds and infiltrates abdominal organs (viscera), such as the colon, small intestine, pancreas, and liver. Abdominal visceral fat is a very different kind of fat, a hotbed of inflammation: View it under a microscope and you will see that this fat is, itself, infiltrated with inflammatory cells. Sample the blood draining from abdominal visceral fat, such as blood drained by the portal venous system from the GI tract to the liver, and you will measure high levels of inflammatory proteins that are exported first to the liver, then on to other parts of the body.[3,4]

Abdominal visceral fat is therefore the number one most powerful source for body-wide inflammation that adds further to weight gain in visceral fat. Inflammation drives resistance to the hormone insulin, causing the pancreas to release far greater amounts to compensate, a response that further expands abdominal visceral fat accumulation. Abdominal visceral fat also leads to distortions in sex hormones, increasing estrogen levels in females, for instance, that increase risk for breast cancer. In males, it increases estrogen and reduces testosterone levels, causing passive social behavior that impairs the ability to deal with stress, and also stimulates growth of male breasts (gynecomastia) and loss of muscle. Yes, abdominal visceral fat is an aesthetic and self-esteem issue, but it is also a serious health issue. Subcutaneous and abdominal visceral fat behave differently, respond to different signals, release different factors into the bloodstream, and have very different consequences for health, weight, and body composition.

A TALE OF TWO BODY SHAPES

Isn't fat just fat? Beyond aesthetics, does it really matter where fat accumulates?

Yes, it most definitely does. Let me compare two make-believe females, but both quite real if you were to set out to identify living counterparts, to illustrate the difference that abdominal visceral fat plays in different body shapes even when the BMI of the two are identical. Then, let's compare two males, likewise with the same BMI but with different body shapes and metabolic patterns.

With the ladies, we'll call one "Julie" and the other "Rachel." Let's start with a level playing field: Julie and Rachel are both 45 years old, both approaching menopause but still premenopausal and experiencing menstrual cycles. Each vaginally delivered two children while in their twenties and thirties, both stand 5 feet 5 inches in height, weigh 180 pounds, and thereby have a BMI of 30. Over the past several years, both women have gradually gained weight, also leapfrogging additional weight during pregnancy, followed by failure to lose the weight after term deliveries. And, over the past several years, both lament that weight gain seems to occur more readily, even when they exercise more, skip meals, or restrict calories. Hopping from Pilates to Zumba classes to yoga to hours on the treadmill—none of it seemed to make a difference.

They are shaped differently—Julie has more of a pear-shaped (gynoid) body configuration, while Rachel has the apple-shaped (android) configuration. (Yes, it can happen in premenopausal females, as well as postmenopausal.) For the sake of argument, let's assume that Julie is almost all pear and Rachel is almost completely an apple. If we were to draw their blood and other measures, we would see something like:

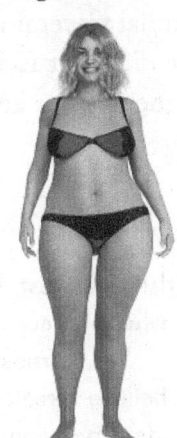

Julie
Blood pressure 104/70
Cholesterol panel:
Total cholesterol 220 mg/dl
LDL cholesterol 148 mg/dl
HDL cholesterol 56 mg/dl
Triglycerides 78 mg/dl
Fasting blood glucose 90 mg/dl
HbA1c 5.2%
C-reactive protein 1.5 mg/dl

Despite her weight and BMI, Julie has normal blood pressure, mostly favorable cholesterol and blood sugar values, and is at relatively low risk for such common conditions as cardiovascular disease, dementia, and breast and other cancers. (Ideal fasting blood glucose is 60–90 mg/dl, while ideal HbA1c is ≤5.0%.) Despite the excess weight, Julie does not have insulin resistance nor increased measures of inflammation (C-reactive protein), as her excess weight is not concentrated in abdominal visceral fat but is mostly subcutaneous fat in the lower half of her body.

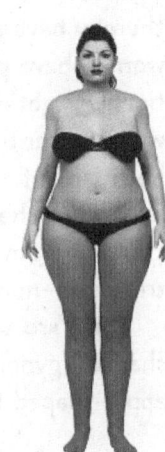

Rachel
Blood pressure 138/84
Cholesterol panel:
Total cholesterol 240 mg/dl
LDL cholesterol 162 mg/dl
HDL cholesterol 40 mg/dl
Triglycerides 190 mg/dl
Fasting blood glucose 112 mg/dl
HbA1c 5.9%
C-reactive protein 3.0 mg/dl

Rachel, whose fat is mostly concentrated in the abdomen, is prediabetic (HbA1c of ≥5.7%), has increased risk for cardiovascular disease, increased risk for cognitive impairment and dementia, and increased risk for breast and other cancers. She has increased insulin resistance and measures of inflammation, suggesting that much of her abdominal fat is intra-abdominal, not subcutaneous. Rachel is more likely to have weaker muscles infiltrated by fat, as well as fat in her knees and hips that accelerates deterioration of joint cartilage, and fat surrounding her heart's (coronary) arteries, adding to her risk for heart disease.

Two females, same age, same premenopausal status, same BMI, but very different distributions of shape, body fat, and thereby health consequences. A number of factors are at work in creating these differences. Rachel, for instance, more likely follows a diet overloaded in carbohydrates and sugars, may have experienced prolonged stress that raised her cortisol levels that encouraged abdominal fat growth, and may also be more genetically susceptible to this fat distribution. Despite their similarities, their health futures are very different. They will also respond differently to various weight-loss maneuvers. Rachel, for example, will respond in an exaggerated way to strategies that specifically target such phenomena as insulin resistance and inflammation. She would benefit by following efforts that specifically target abdominal visceral fat first, preserve or increase muscle that accelerates the weight-loss process, and will move the entire panel of unfavorable blood measures back to looking more like Julie's, thereby reducing or eliminating risk for all the common health conditions mentioned.

But it's not all roses for Julie either. Over the years, despite the metabolic advantages that she enjoys with her pear-shaped fat distribution, she will gradually transition in both appearance and metabolic factors to look more like Rachel, developing more abdominal visceral fat and losing muscle, and will, over time, also come to mirror Rachel's abnormal metabolic markers. She will experience such adverse effects later in life and thereby experience serious health consequences more toward her sixties, seventies, and onward, whereas Rachel experiences them decades earlier. Efforts that Julie makes today, while not yielding the same magnitude of advantages as they do for Rachel, will therefore help prevent future deterioration.

Beyond the differences in fat distribution, both women also lose muscle, due to aging alone. It means that, over time, they have less and less control over their basal metabolic rate (BMR), gaining fat weight, subcutaneous and visceral, even if they reduce calorie intake. So it is important to recognize that the challenge is not calorie intake; it's specifically targeting abdominal visceral fat, restoring muscle mass lost with aging, and cutting calories, an approach that we shall pursue through the ideas presented in SUPER Body.

Let's now consider two men, Jeff and Sam. Unlike the ladies, Jeff and Sam start with a BMI of 27, just a little above a BMI of 25, the value generally regarded as normal or ideal.

Both men are 48 years old, both are moderately active and engage in exercise three or four times per week, mostly walking, biking, and some resistance exercise, as well as the occasional round of golf or tennis. Both had body composition measured using a body composition (bioimpedance) scale. The device reveals that Jeff has 19 percent fat and 59 kg (118 lbs) of muscle, while Sam has 30 percent fat and 45 kg (99 lbs) of muscle, all at the same BMI.

Jeff
Blood pressure 128/80
Cholesterol panel:
Total cholesterol 220 mg/dl
LDL cholesterol 142 mg/dl
HDL cholesterol 50 mg/dl
Triglycerides 140 mg/dl
Fasting blood glucose 98 mg/dl
HbA1c 5.3%
C-reactive protein 1.0 mg/dl

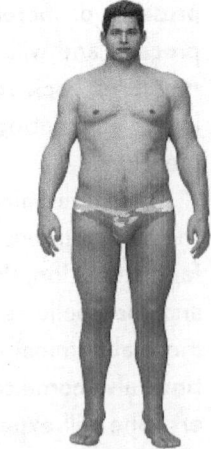

Consistent with fairly favorable fat percentage and muscle mass, Jeff is in pretty good (though not ideal) metabolic shape at a BMI of 27.

Sam
Blood pressure 150/88
Cholesterol panel:
Total cholesterol 198 mg/dl
LDL cholesterol 162 mg/dl
HDL cholesterol 35 mg/dl
Triglycerides 240 mg/dl
Fasting blood glucose 112 mg/dl
HbA1c 5.9%
C-reactive protein 3.0 mg/dl

At the same BMI, Sam is hypertensive and has HDL cholesterol and triglycerides that put him at higher risk of cardiovascular disease. (I disregard the widely used LDL cholesterol as being an invalid and unreliable index of cardiovascular risk, a conversation for another time. But, by conventional standards, Sam has greater risk posed by the higher LDL cholesterol.) His blood sugar measures, fasting glucose, and HbA1c place Sam in the prediabetic range, while there is increased inflammation status as revealed by the high C-reactive protein.

If Sam weighed himself using a bioimpedance device that scored visceral fat (most devices do not provide an actual weight of visceral fat but provide a "score"), he would score high. In other words, despite the appearance of a favorable BMI, Sam's body shape and composition with excessive abdominal fat and lack of muscle puts him at higher risk for numerous health conditions.

Here we have two men with the same BMI but different body shapes and compositions, different metabolic situations with varying risk for health conditions, one low and one high. We could label Sam as being so-called skinny fat; that is, appearing outwardly slender but, due to excessive abdominal visceral fat, he is metabolically obese. You can therefore

appreciate that a method, such as calorie reduction, that preferentially targets loss of subcutaneous fat would not be ideal
and would not yield full benefit. You can also appreciate that
Sam will be impaired in his ability to lose abdominal visceral fat
due to his lack of muscle that thereby slows his metabolic rate,
a phenomenon that is worsened should he try to lose weight
by reducing calories. None of this is factored into conventional
notions of losing weight.

BLAME WHERE BLAME IS DUE

Obesity per se is therefore not the problem; fat in the abdomen that
surrounds abdominal organs, abdominal visceral fat, is the source of
nearly all the health consequences associated with carrying excess
weight. Unless we take specific action, the situation worsens with each
passing year as we experience increased visceral fat and lose muscle.

Over the past two decades, as the expanding bodies of many struggle to find new places to store excess fat, something called ectopic fat
has also made a debut, fat found in peculiar locations, such as the liver,
pancreas, kidneys, knees, hips, heart—places where accumulated fat
significantly accelerates disease. Fat surrounding the organs is particularly dangerous to your health in that it can damage those organs
and diminish how they function. For example, ectopic fat that accumulates in the knees inflames knee cartilage, accelerating the disinte-
gration of cartilage that leads to bone-on-bone arthritis. Ectopic fat in
the pancreas damages the beta cells that produce insulin, converting a
type 2 diabetic into a type 1 diabetic dependent on insulin injections,
a development for which there is no turning back. Ectopic fat in the
kidney compresses the arteries and veins entering and leaving the kidney, which leads to hypertension and kidney disease. Fat sitting on the
surface of the heart, called epicardial fat, accelerates the development
of atherosclerosis in the heart's arteries, bringing a person closer to a
heart attack, such procedures as stent implantation or bypass surgery,

and sudden cardiac death. No, this is not just a cosmetic issue; it's a very serious issue for health.[5]

If abdominal and ectopic fat are the source of nearly all problems associated with obesity, shouldn't we focus our efforts on these forms of fat and not on the fat in the buttocks, thighs, arms, or other subcutaneous fat depots? If we target abdominal visceral fat first, many of the factors driving unhealthy weight gain unravel, making fat loss from *all* body locales easier and easier, including that from subcutaneous fat. Yet all conventional efforts at weight loss preferentially target subcutaneous, not abdominal, fat. Let me repeat that idea for emphasis: Conventional methods of weight loss preferentially target more benign subcutaneous fat, not abdominal visceral fat, and therefore fail to focus on correcting the source of insulin resistance and inflammation that drive weight gain.[6]

Someone who is insulin resistant has much higher—often ten- or a hundredfold higher—levels of insulin, a hormone that drives deposition of abdominal fat that, in turn, amplifies inflammation, all of which further fans the flames of insulin resistance, a dangerously vicious cycle that, if conventional approaches continue, ensures continual expansion of abdominal fat and loss of muscle. Conventional weight-loss efforts, whether diet, pharmaceuticals, or bariatric procedures, are therefore slower and less effective in improving body shape and composition, and also do not provide the full range of benefits that develop when you preferentially target abdominal visceral and ectopic fat first.

THE PONZI SCHEME OF WEIGHT LOSS

Surely you've encountered headlines reporting on the many Ponzi schemes operating in modern society. They involve life insurance, real estate, investments—but it's all the same: promising high financial returns by taking new money from unwitting investors to pay off old, with no real investments involved, just robbing Peter to pay Paul. The schemes of Bernie Madoff, Sam Bankman-Fried, and others yield big up-front profits for the scam artist in the form of mansions, Bentleys, and diamond jewelry until whistleblowers or legal authorities expose the fraud.

Conventional approaches to weight loss are not that different: health and weight-loss Ponzi schemes that yield up-front profits but eventually collapse. Whether some version of "move more, eat less," pharmaceutical agents, or bariatric procedures, they are all variations on the same theme: reducing calories to fund your initial "investment."

It could be one of the countless programs or smartphone apps to help identify appetite triggers, or count points, or provide ready-made meals—all aim to reduce intake of calories. We could administer pharmaceuticals that, along with nausea, vomiting, and risk for pancreatitis and bowel obstruction, turn off desire for food, causing the user to take in fewer calories. Or it could involve a bariatric procedure, such as gastric bypass or a lap-band, which reduces stomach volume, yielding satiety with fewer calories. But they all rely on the same strategy of causing users to consume less food and thereby fewer calories.

The problem with reducing calories, regardless of the method used, is that *it inevitably causes loss of muscle*. Approximately 25 percent of all weight lost is muscle.[7] Say you lose 40 pounds by injecting yourself with the newest GLP-1 agonist drug. Of those 40 pounds, 10 or more pounds lost is muscle. Imagine 10 pounds of ground beef on your kitchen table—that's a lot of muscle. You stop the drug and promptly regain around 32 or more pounds, nearly all of which is fat, mostly abdominal visceral fat, with very little return of muscle. You now have more fat than when you started and are at *greater* risk for heart disease, stroke, type 2 diabetes, dementia, breast cancer, and other diseases than you were at the start, all due to the loss of muscle.[8] In the Ponzi scheme of conventional weight loss, you eventually pay the price. Not only are you now worse off financially, but you are also closer to emotional and metabolic bankruptcy. Of course, if your gastric bypass or lap-band fails to maintain your slender figure, the doctor has their prescription pad ready to prescribe a weight-loss drug, or makes a recommendation to consult with a dietitian on how to reduce calories and fat. Reducing calorie intake is, at so many levels, an ill-fated scheme little different from the scamster who pockets your well-earned retirement money.

Carl, 59

"I LOST WEIGHT USING CALORIE RESTRICTION AND EXERCISE. I was having a hard time maintaining the weight loss. It seemed that every time I put anything into my mouth, I would gain a half a pound or a pound or two. I had also lost a lot of muscle mass and looked emaciated. Some even said I looked like I was sick. I was also having a hard time getting rid of the visceral fat around my belly.

"I came across Dr. Davis's program while I was researching sustainable weight loss. I gained weight at first and I was a little concerned, but I think it was my body resetting my metabolism. The immediate effects were definitely connected to bowel flora and those results have been amazing. I continued the same workout routine that I was doing prior (actually less) but this time the results were different. My muscle mass increased over an inch on my biceps, neck, calves and thighs (I gained a total of 6 lbs of muscle), while my belly (visceral fat) decreased by 4 inches. I also noticed that I wasn't starving like I was on the other diet and actually ate almost double the calories per day. My stamina has increased and my mind is clearer than it's been since my twenties. (I'm 59.) I feel more empathy towards others and even find myself caring more for people in general."

All calorie-reducing strategies that target subcutaneous fat make weight *regain* inevitable, a booby trap that sets you up for long-term failure from the start, since the processes that caused weight in the first place—insulin resistance and inflammation—are not addressed by preferentially losing subcutaneous fat.

What if you could specifically target loss of abdominal visceral fat without reducing calories, thereby improving the process of insulin resistance that originates with visceral fat and reducing levels of fat-expanding insulin, accelerating loss of subcutaneous fat while preserving or even increasing muscle mass that gives you control over metabolic rate? You would lose weight from all fat compartments, but especially abdominal visceral fat, and not be exposed to risk for regaining the weight. Isn't that a smarter path? But is it possible? It absolutely is possible and involves no calorie-cutting, no hunger, no obsessing about food, no counting points, no loss of muscle and thereby no regain of lost weight, no need to outlay huge sums of money, no need for your health insurer to approve the process. Don't worry, loss of subcutaneous fat will follow—we just don't start there.

And, as a bonus, the methods I shall be sharing also yield effects such as smoother skin with less wrinkles, better sleep, increased libido, enhanced immune response, and improved well-being. Getting thinner is only the beginning—you can also enjoy better health, restored youthfulness, and better relationships. In short, you can be a better human being, all bulges in their proper place.

GLP-1 AGONISTS: THE $10 BILLION WEIGHT-LOSS DISASTER

The release of GLP-1 agonist weight-loss drugs over the past few years have represented an unprecedented financial windfall for the pharmaceutical industry. Doctors have declared these drugs to be a "breakthrough" for weight loss, "lifesavers," even "magical." Celebrities gush at their weight-loss results, showing off their newfound slenderness in tight outfits. None of them recognizes that these endorsements are sending people on a path of health-care and financial disaster.

As we've discussed, yes, you can indeed lose a substantial quantity of weight with these drugs, but weight regain is inevitable when the drug is stopped. You have a choice: Accept the weight regain that is mostly fat, not muscle, when the drugs are stopped, thereby leaving you unhealthier—more insulin resistant, more likely prediabetic or diabetic than before, with increased risk for heart disease, cancer, and cognitive impairment—than when you started. Or stay on the drugs for a lifetime, shelling out $1,000 to $1,500 every month, $120,000 to $180,000 over a decade, provided they don't raise the price. The fundamental means by which these drugs work—reduction in calorie intake—has been proven to result in long-term failure and weight regain when the drugs are stopped. They are the perfect example of a quick "fix" that leads to long-term failure.

To illustrate, let's take Betsy: 240 pounds, around 110 pounds overweight, with the start of high blood sugar, high blood pressure, fatty liver, and knee arthritis, as well as low self-esteem, having to shop in the plus-size aisle and unable to wear clothes she loved from just a few years earlier. Her doctor prescribes a GLP-1 agonist, warning her about side effects. Still, she accepts the prescription. Over a year, Betsy loses 40 pounds, now down to 200 pounds—still overweight, but less so, an experience that has cost her thousands of dollars. Twenty-five percent of the weight lost, or 10 pounds, caused her basal metabolic rate (BMR) to decrease. Unable to sustain this expense indefinitely, she stops the injections. Despite limiting calorie intake, sometimes below 1,200 calories per day, and struggling with incessant cravings and food obsessions, she regains 32 pounds, most of it as fat around her waist. Her doctor now tells her she is prediabetic and that her hypertension and fatty liver have returned. And her knees hurt worse than ever. She is now demoralized and poorer, with greater risk for multiple chronic diseases than she was at the start of this misadventure and likely shortening her life by several years.[9] Betsy will also likely notice that she looks ten or twenty years older, a phenomenon some have labeled "Ozempic face," the sagging, deep wrinkles that develop due to GLP-1 agonist's preferential loss of subcutaneous fat, including that in the face, and loss of facial muscle. (By the way, I shall discuss later how the strategies advocated in SUPER Body do not generate the age-accelerating Ozempic face but achieve the opposite: preservation of facial muscles, reduction of skin wrinkles, and restoration of youthful facial features.) Temporarily more slender, but appearing much older, with deteriorating health after their cessation—such is the price of this deeply flawed class of drugs.

Someone like Betsy therefore has a choice: Remain on the drug forever with continued exposure to cost and side effects, or go off the drug and accept that, despite enjoying a year or so of slenderness, weight will rebound. In reality, Betsy has no good choices, as the initial choices she made—advocated by her doctor—were not good choices in the first place but destined to fail from the start.

Read a marketing pitch for a weight-loss program, or the warnings of side effects from a weight-loss drug, or receive the urgings of your doctor to undergo a bariatric procedure, and you will not encounter any mention of the inevitable loss of muscle that all these methods entail. That is a big oversight. But loss of muscle provoked by all these weight-loss approaches is the land mine planted that will eventually explode, putting you back where you started and actually less healthy, with more abdominal fat, less muscle, and reduced BMR, leaving you feeling hopeless.

THE NOT-SO-GLOWING TRACK RECORD OF BARIATRIC PROCEDURES

Given the profound inadequacies of pharmaceutical solutions to weight and misplaced bulges, doctors then resort to bariatric procedures as the ultimate gold standard, a surgical means of circumventing excessive calorie intake to lose weight. Proponents boast about the long-term success in losing and maintaining weight loss. While there can indeed be significant weight loss, many people undergoing these procedures experience a peculiar list of long-term health problems rarely mentioned in sales pitches from doctors and clinics offering them. This has become big business, now a $2-billion-per-year enterprise with many gastroenterologists and general surgeons busy making people's stomach volumes smaller.

But are the glowing reports true?

Bariatric procedures are nowadays typically performed laparoscopically (i.e., via a scope inserted through a puncture in the abdominal wall) or robotically (also through a small puncture). The various versions of weight-loss surgery have also undergone refinements in recent years, allowing faster recovery and fewer complications. It is also true that, because of the weight lost up front, there will be improvements in various weight-sensitive biomarkers, such as blood sugar, blood pressure, and such conditions as type 2 diabetes and sleep apnea. Mainstream opinion is that these procedures are so safe and effective that the American Academy of Pediatrics has endorsed these procedures for children.[10] So, what is there not to like?

There are issues that can be easily remedied, especially nutritional deficiencies of iron, vitamin B_{12}, folate, and other nutrients, and the frequent development of gallstones that typically require gallbladder removal. There is also the development of small intestinal bacterial overgrowth (SIBO) in about 50 percent of people who have undergone one of these procedures, likely due to the reduction in stomach acid that results.[11] (Stomach acid is an effective barrier to the descent of microbes from the mouth and the ascent of fecal microbes, allowing the stomach and small intestine to become colonized with these invading microbes. It's a situation with broad implications for health that include increased weight regain, increased risk for type 2 diabetes, heart disease, cognitive decline, and others. Later in the book, I shall discuss this issue further.) Taken at face value, however, the reports are glowing: substantial weight loss, minimal mortality of a fraction of 1 percent, or fewer than 1 in 1,000.[12]

The reporting on the outcomes of bariatric procedures is, in many ways, a microcosm that reflects much of what is wrong with health care in general: studies performed by physicians compensated generously by companies that manufacture the equipment required to perform the procedures, over-the-top successes reported that do not seem to jive with real-world experience, and selective underreporting of serious complications including need for reoperation, critical illness, and death. If death occurs from complications of the procedure in only 1 in 1,000 people, of the 260,000 procedures performed in 2021 in the United States, there were only 260 deaths.[13,14] If true, this would be an admirable record, given the risks of operative procedures in general. But in many instances, follow-up after a procedure is dismal, the fate of the majority of people lost, meaning that many complications are simply not counted.

Because of the inadequacies of the reporting process, we only get hints that something worse is going on. Include among the recent deaths Lisa Marie Presley, daughter of Elvis Presley, who died at age fifty-four of intestinal adhesions several years after her gastric bypass. (Intestinal adhesions are an accompaniment of any procedure in which the intestines have been surgically manipulated, an effect that can cause constrictions and thereby catastrophic obstruction of the passage of digestive material down the GI tract.) One of the most concerning issues in the years after a bariatric procedure is the three- to fourfold increase in suicide, and many more attempted suicides.[15]

Proponents of bariatric procedures—including most physicians who perform such procedures—point out that, without such procedures, obese people die more than ten years earlier, often much more, than non-obese people, and that weight loss achieved through a procedure adds ten or more years to life span. If you were desperate with obesity, disappointed with endless nonprocedural efforts to find solutions, then it seems to be a reasonable trade-off: Have the procedure and accept some risk. But this isn't the best question to ask. Let's ask instead: What if a smarter approach were adopted to not just achieve fat loss but specifically target abdominal visceral fat while preserving muscle mass using nonsurgical methods that therefore do not risk hemorrhage, infection, nutritional deficiencies, intestinal adhesions, suicide, and other postoperative complications? And we also take steps to increase muscle and thereby BMR?

It is, undoubtedly, a murky situation. Obese people have more than excess fat to contend with. They are also more likely to have diabetes, heart disease, higher levels of inflammation, and other health conditions, overt or hidden, that can add to a stormy postprocedural course. There are also reports of unexpected complications of the procedure, such as choking from regurgitated stomach contents, intractable vomiting, drug and alcohol abuse, various forms of neuropathy, frequent episodes of hypoglycemia, and, of course, suicide.[16-21] Should a woman of childbearing age undergo a bariatric procedure and then get pregnant, there is a high likelihood of complications that result in maternal or fetal death.[22] In other words, life after a bariatric procedure is not characterized as healthy slenderness, but a life filled with peculiar complications that are not fully understood. The many accounts of such complications call into question the rosy picture painted by available studies, a likely consequence of underreporting by sources with a stake in reporting on the safety of these procedures. Such exaggerated claims of benefit are not unique to bariatric procedures, by the way, but plague the health-care industry in general. Look at the common and widespread prescription of statin drugs to reduce cholesterol and risk for cardiovascular disease, for example. Claims are typically made that such drugs reduce cardiovascular risk by 36 to 55 percent, when the reality is that these drugs hardly reduce risk at all but have brought hundreds of billions of dollars in revenue to the pharmaceutical industry.[23]

As with all other forms of caloric reduction, bariatric procedures, such as gastric bypass, suffer from similar issues of preferential loss of subcutaneous fat and long-term weight regain due to loss of muscle.[6,7] Thinner in the beginning, yes, but more prone to numerous diseases and weight regain over time.

By following the ideas shared in this book, you will experience no surgical incision, not have to battle with your health insurance plan, and not risk postoperative complications, nor will you experience long-term health problems associated with an unnatural rerouting of your stomach contents.

THE SHAPE OF THINGS TO COME

It's time to reject all the messaging you've received over the years that essentially guarantees failure, even after initially positive results. Forget the advice to "cut your fat, eat more healthy whole grains"; "move more, eat less"; "everything in moderation"—all the false mantras that, in truth, result in distortions of shape and body composition, as well as health. Reject conventional "wisdom" and replace it with strategies that not only result in loss of fat weight, especially from abdominal visceral fat, but also restore lost muscle and thereby maintain or increase BMR. We thereby shrink the various abnormal bulges and protuberances while restoring youthful contours. You will be able to track a reduction in waist circumference, followed by reduced collections of subcutaneous fat distributed throughout, even noticing that your arms, shoulders, and thighs are firmer. You will even likely experience a change in facial contours with less around-the-eyes puffiness, less jowly cheeks, receding double chin, and firmer facial muscles.

Before we go on to discuss the various factors that allow you to change course, let's make sure that you understand all that goes haywire when you adopt conventional advice. That way, you will understand with crystal clarity why such strategies do not work. This will help steer you in the direction of strategies that really do work, even if they seem unfamiliar or counterintuitive.

2

EAT TO YOUR GENETIC CODE

I F OBESITY AND THE VARIOUS DISTORTIONS OF BODY SHAPE that humans experience are creations of modern habits, phenomena not preprogrammed into the human genetic code, does this realization provide insight into how to undo the entire body composition mess?

Look at human hunter-gatherers in the Brazilian rainforest or natives of the Tanzanian savannah or jungles of New Guinea: They do not struggle with obesity or irregular body shapes. Look at animals in the wild—any bobcat, alligator, or salmon: no obesity. (Revealingly, dogs and cats that we have domesticated into our homes show the same perverse pattern of unprecedented weight gain as humans.) Being overweight or obese is not entirely new to "civilized" populations, as there have been occasional people struggling with weight all throughout history. There was a time, for instance, when "Rubenesque" referred to a soft, round female form and was considered beautiful and desirable; and a "portly" gentleman was considered respected and successful. But in no previous time in human history have struggles with weight and body composition been as widespread and suffered to the severe degree that we, as modern people, struggle with. Health and youthful body contours are actually programmed in your genetic code, a virtual blueprint, but it is a code we have essentially ignored and paid the body composition price.

What do hunter-gatherer humans and wild animals have that we don't have? A number of crucial factors, all of which help determine shape and body composition. Some of these factors are dietary, some are environmental, and others are microbial (dependent on microbes dwelling in the gastrointestinal [GI] tract). Reliance on commercial processed foods, rather than whole foods in their natural state, has played a major role. The modern aversion to consuming organ meats, such as brain, tongue, and heart, generate deficiencies in factors that substantially affect body composition. Loss of specific GI microbes means that we do without the considerable advantages they provide in shaping body composition. Advice to "move more, eat less" or "eat many small meals every two hours" can completely miss the mark on how to restore ideal shape and body composition. But, as you will learn in this book, by rejecting conventional notions of weight control, then embracing factors that should have been part of your life all along, you can seize back control over the distribution of fat, muscle, and body contours. Don't worry: Despite the talk of consuming organ meats, you will not have to feast on pancreas and tongue to succeed at this lifestyle.

In this chapter, we'll tee up the logic that serves as the basis for the eating style discussed in greater detail later in the book. Let's begin by considering the modern practices that are to blame for distorting modern shapes and body composition, mistakes that we can remedy.

"YOU LIVE ONLY ONCE," "EVERYTHING IN MODERATION," AND OTHER DISASTROUS ADVICE

Advising Americans to cut fat and cholesterol from the diet is just another in a long series of blunders. Numerous examples of misguided advice, now largely abandoned as useless or harmful, fill the cemetery of outdated dietary guidelines. Remember how we were urged to replace butter with margarine? This led to a huge health disaster as margarine is largely a trans fat–based product, made by bubbling hydrogen gas through liquid oil at high temperature to convert liquid to solid (hydrogenation), estimated to have been responsible for as many as fifty thousand premature deaths per year before legislative action was taken to limit their use in processed foods.[1,2]

Health organizations that purport to deliver health messages jumped on the low-fat, low-cholesterol bandwagon. Since 1995, a number of foods most of us would deem unhealthy have proudly borne the American Heart Association (AHA) "Heart-Check" stamp of approval—for instance, Pop-Tarts, Cocoa Puffs, Count Chocula, and Berry Berry Kix. Quaker Instant Oatmeal Apples & Cinnamon enjoyed the AHA's endorsement for many years, despite the fact that each serving contains the equivalent of over 11 teaspoons of sugar (even more in older versions of the product), with ingredients that included sugar, corn syrup, flaked corn, and partially hydrogenated cottonseed oil. The American Diabetes Association (ADA), for many years, has advocated high intake of carbohydrates and low intake of fat, despite the well-established fact that carbohydrates are the principal driver of high blood sugars. ADA dietary advice was designed more to prevent hypoglycemia (low blood sugar) when diabetes medications, such as insulin, were introduced; such a diet was not intended to reverse the disease or its causes, nor reduce its complications. Even today, educational material from the ADA asks: "If you have type 2 diabetes and your doctor says you need to start using insulin, does it mean you're failing to take care of your diabetes properly?" Their response: "Using insulin to get blood glucose levels to a healthy level is a good thing, not a bad one," essentially ignoring the evidence that tells us that initiating injectable insulin is the start of a rapid downward spiral in health, accelerating weight gain, increasing difficulty controlling blood sugar, and bringing the user closer to organ complications, such as blindness, heart disease, and kidney failure.[3,4]

The resultant increase in carbohydrate and sugar ingestion and reduction of fats by Americans also caused prediabetes and type 2 diabetes to develop in half the US population, with many more showing insulin resistance that leads over time to these conditions, an unprecedented disaster.[5] Not only is insulin resistance the fundamental process that puts us at increased risk for coronary heart disease, type 2 diabetes, weight gain, dementia, and other conditions, it is also a situation that leads to sodium retention by the kidneys.[6] (This is a situation that reverses with the strategies articulated in *SUPER Body*. During Week 1, as instructed in this book, you will reverse insulin resistance, and thereby sodium retention that was causing you to retain large quantities of water weight [inflammatory edema].) Such agencies as the FDA and most doctors urge everyone to reduce salt intake, blaming salt, rather than sodium-retaining insulin resistance, for high blood pressure and increased cardiovascular risk. By mistakenly doing so, they not only demonized the wrong culprit but also forgot that iodized salt is the main source of iodine for most Americans and that increased consumption of iodized salt was the agency's original advice. Reduced reliance on iodized salt has led to a reappearance of thyroid dysfunction, goiters (enlarged thyroid glands on the neck), and hypothyroidism (low levels of thyroid hormone), situations reminiscent of life prior to the introduction of iodized salt in 1924, when iodine deficiency was epidemic. This adds yet another factor causing weight gain and type 2 diabetes. Yes: Insulin resistance, increased risk for multiple modern diseases, iodine deficiency, and thyroid dysfunction, all contributing to weight gain and distortions of shape and body composition, are all caused or worsened by conventional dietary advice.[7]

Some of the most troubling advice has come from the Academy of Nutrition and Dietetics (AND), the organization that educates and certifies dietitians and nutritionists, efforts largely supported by generous donations from the food and pharmaceutical industries. AND takes the stand that all foods—soft drinks, candy bars, sugary breakfast cereals, high-fructose corn syrup–containing snacks, etc.—fit into a healthy lifestyle, provided you manage calories and exercise. For instance, a recent AND position statement declares: "All foods can fit within this pattern if consumed in moderation with appropriate portion size and combined with physical activity."[8] In other words, go ahead and have that can of sugary soda or slice of pie, but you may have to exercise for an additional thirty minutes or cut back on other calorie sources to compensate, a position that completely ignores the science that tells us that numerous issues are caused by such unsophisticated advice. Consumption of sugars, for instance, provokes formation of lipoproteins in the bloodstream that lead to heart disease, causes irreversible glycation (glucose modification of proteins) in the brain that contributes to risk for cognitive decline, and unfavorably alters gastrointestinal bowel flora—effects that cannot be undone by a bit of exercise or reducing other caloric sources.

These are just some examples. Over and over again, dietary guidelines and conventional dietary advice got it wrong, delivering advice to Americans that has been not just ineffective but dangerous, not uncommonly causing or worsening diseases they were intended to prevent. The low-fat, low-cholesterol message, coupled with the proliferation of processed and ultraprocessed foods, has not only contributed to the epidemics of obesity and type 2 diabetes. It also led to deficiencies of several important nutrients that play roles in shape and body composition.

Add collagen, hyaluronic acid, and carotenoids to the list of dietary casualties, factors lost in the diet of modern people due to ill-conceived dietary advice. Few people nowadays include animal-sourced tripe (stomach), intestines, skin, or heart in their daily diet. Many people, in fact, make efforts to buy such foods as boneless, skinless chicken breast, lacking the collagen content of bones and absent the rich hyaluronic acid content of the skin. Rather than a salad of kale, spinach, and dandelion greens containing abundant carotenoids, most people now opt for nachos with cheese.

The solution: Reject advice to reduce fat and cholesterol, embrace organ meats (or their equivalents) and other sources of these nutrients, and return to real, whole foods.

JUST ADD WATER, READY-TO-EAT, AND PRIZE INSIDE!

It was only a century ago that having chicken for dinner meant getting one from your chicken coop or barn, defeathering and butchering it yourself before cooking it. If you wanted to feed your family green beans or beets, you would harvest them from your garden. You were

as close to the source of your food as your backyard or the family farm
down the road.

The emergence of the processed food industry changed all that.
Methods once used to ensure survival through tough winter months
and to keep food from spoiling, practices such as canning, fermentation, and curing meats in open air, all fell by the wayside. Modern food
processing was celebrated for the convenience it provided, a way to
slash the amount of time a traditional housewife might devote to preparing and cooking food. No need to do anything the hard way—there
was mac and cheese in a box, premade breakfast cereals, ice pops to
snack on. Microwaveable dinners became a staple—no more baking
from scratch—breakfast became as quick and easy as popping a "tart"
in the toaster. Order up a feast delivered by a ride-hailing app with a
few taps on your smartphone and you'll have an instant meal, no mention of whether the food is organic, was cooked in unhealthy oils, or
contains a long list of additives.

As perverse as these foods are, food processing more recently has
been taken to an absurd extreme. Think: genetically modified corn
laden with glyphosate, the herbicide that kills weeds but not corn, but
also kills beneficial microbes in your GI tract because of its antibiotic
properties. Or modern wheat that is the result of thousands of genetic
experiments to alter its properties, yielding a plant that looks nothing like its natural predecessors and provokes a wide range of peculiar
effects on humans who unwittingly consume it. Food manufacturers
have added such ingredients as polysorbate 80 or carboxymethylcellulose that, yes, keep ice cream mixed when thawed and refrozen or
tertiary butylhydroquinone that prolongs the shelf life of crackers,
synthetic additives that also provoke inflammation in the consumer,
kill beneficial GI microbes, and increase insulin resistance that leads to
weight gain and distortions of body composition and triggers mental
and emotional disturbances. Emulsifying agents, mixing agents such
as carrageenan and gellan gum, artificial colorings, and, of course, the
unprecedented quantities of sugars, all conspire to introduce effects
that grow abdominal fat as well as cultivate insulin resistance and

inflammation, expanding the various bulges and protuberances that you see all around you.[9,10] You may push the plate away or add another thirty minutes to your exercise routine, but by engaging in the standard American diet, you have guaranteed your own failure in taking command over body composition.

Food manufacturers are also experts at identifying ingredients that amplify cravings, creating a class of so-called ultraprocessed foods that also add to weight gain and obesity.[11] You will quickly recognize the powdered cheese, white flour, high-fructose corn syrup, cornstarch, and tablespoons of sugar that dominate the ingredient list in the majority of ultraprocessed foods. And, let's face it, the marketing of these products to consumers is very effective, especially when directed toward children and lower-income groups. Just as tobacco manufacturers famously targeted teenagers and people in lower socio-economic groups, so has the food industry exerted predatory marketing pitches on those most vulnerable—and it works. It is not uncommon for children, for instance, to obtain half or more of their calories from ultraprocessed foods, such as frozen pizza, soft drinks, and chips, habits that cultivate expansion of abdominal visceral fat.[12] Even mature adults with a lifetime of experience and dietary trials and errors are not immune. A recent survey of adults ages fifty to eighty years, revealed that 44 percent experienced addictive behavior toward one or more ultraprocessed foods, many admitting to dealing with intense cravings and withdrawal phenomena.[13] You will rarely see TV, magazine, or social media ads for extra-virgin olive oil, salmon, or eggs. There will be no Hollywood spokesperson for organ meats or celebrity rock star promoting the benefits of butter. But you will see no shortage of pitches for chips, fast foods, or soft drinks.

Modern processed and ultraprocessed foods are therefore a shape and body composition nightmare, essentially ensuring that you expand visceral fat stores and amplify insulin resistance and inflammation, cultivating bulges, lumps, and other body distortions starting as early as childhood.

LESSONS LEARNED FROM THE WORLDWIDE WHEAT BELLY EXPERIENCE

The arguments I provided in my *Wheat Belly* books did not involve cutting calories. The whole adventure began with my efforts to eliminate one of the real causes of heart disease: small LDL particles—not LDL cholesterol, an outdated concept that should have been discarded decades ago. Although they sound somewhat alike, they are worlds apart. Small LDL particles persist for five to seven days (much longer than the twenty-four hours of benign large LDL particles), are more readily able to enter the walls of arteries, trigger inflammation, are prone to oxidation, and thereby lead to atherosclerosis, the material that causes heart attacks, angina, and sudden cardiac death. LDL cholesterol does not cause heart disease; the concept of LDL cholesterol was meant to be a crude and indirect method to guestimate the number of LDL particles, the actual particles in the bloodstream that cause heart attacks. But you and I can directly measure LDL particles and measure their size and have no need of the outdated and nearly useless LDL cholesterol value.

The only foods that trigger inflammatory, oxidation-prone, adhesive, and oddly persistent small LDL particles? Wheat and other grains, and sugar—not butter, not pork fat, not bacon, not olive oil.[14] Out of frustration with the fact that reducing dietary saturated fat and LDL cholesterol with statin drugs hardly makes a dent in cardiovascular risk, not even close to eliminating the potential for dangerous cardiac events, I asked patients to permanently banish all wheat and other grains and sugars from their diets. Lo and behold, small LDL (measured via a method called nuclear magnetic resonance [NMR]) dropped to the floor. A high-risk starting value of, say, 2,400 nmol/L (particle count per volume) would drop to zero or other very low value, essentially *eliminating* a potent source of cardiovascular risk.

But the elimination of wheat, other grains, and sugar also yielded dramatic improvements in health: relief from skin rashes, reductions in blood sugar sufficient to stop one or more diabetes drugs, drops in blood pressure that necessitated stopping blood pressure medications, reduction or relief of joint pain, and many other unexpected developments. The people adopting this lifestyle watched their waists shrink dramatically while retaining muscle mass. Doing the *opposite* of what most physicians and dietitians advised yielded huge and unexpected health benefits. Over and over again, I watched type 2 diabetics become nondiabetic; people with binge-eating disorder regain control over appetite; and women with polycystic ovary syndrome lose their excessive body hair and hypertension, and become pregnant. And I personally witnessed thousands of people lose their abdominal fat and shrink waist circumference, gaining vigor and strength in the process.

CHRISTIE

"Before starting *Wheat Belly*, I had debilitating ulcerative colitis. I was afraid to leave the house. I would even cancel or avoid family gatherings for fear of not making it to the bathroom in time. It was a very depressing time in my life.

"A friend suggested *Wheat Belly* and I bought the book. My life has changed for the good forever. My gastroenterologist said at my last colonoscopy there isn't even a trace of my ulcerative colitis. He is now advising other patients to go wheat- and grain-free after seeing my success and results. Also, I used to have gum issues and cavities and now my gum health is great and no cavities for many years."

RITA, 76

"After the age of 50 years, my weight seemed to creep on. I tried dieting without success. I'm 5'2" and was miserable at my highest weight of 224 pounds.

"We ladies were going coloring at the local library. A friend had just lost 100 pounds following *Wheat Belly*. Her doctor just took her off insulin shots and she looked amazing. I bought the books and my journey started there. I have learned this way-of-eating is easy. It's all about avoiding wheat, grains, and sugar. My overall health has improved and I have more energy and stamina."

There are a number of reasons that this approach works. Elimination of wheat and other grains:

- Eliminates the highly digestible amylopectin A carbohydrate unique to wheat and other grains that raises blood glucose and thereby insulin, causing abdominal visceral fat to expand.[15] Eating a diet rich in "healthy whole grains" is a little different from a diet filled with sugar-filled candy and desserts. Banishing sources of amylopectin A allows insulin resistance to reverse, thereby allowing you to release the energy stored in abdominal visceral fat. (It also eliminates, by the way, a major factor causing tooth decay, just like table sugar and candy.)

- Eliminates gliadin-derived opioid peptides, which originate with gluten protein and are potent appetite stimulants.[16] Eliminating the source of these opioids puts you in control over appetite and impulse. Hunger is no longer intense and desperate but a soft occasional reminder to eat something. You will lose the impulse to plunder the refrigerator at all hours for something more to eat; you will find yourself satisfied with less food compared to others while eating at restaurants; you will notice that foods you formerly liked, such as a milk chocolate bar or corn chips, are now intolerably and sickeningly sweet or unpalatable. In short, your appetites and impulses revert back to a more natural state.

- We do not restrict fats or oils: There never was solid evidence to prove that saturated fat caused heart disease or that reducing saturated fat reduces risk. We therefore enjoy butter, olive oil, and fatty cuts of meat. Fats are not only important for the delicious and varied tastes of food but also satiating: They keep you satisfied and away from junk foods. Have a grain-free, sugar-free breakfast of eggs and sausage at seven a.m. and you likely won't be hungry until late afternoon, if at all—very different from the insatiable, never satisfied experience of the grain-eating public.

There are other reasons that this *Wheat Belly* approach yielded unexpected and substantial health benefits. But that's it in a nutshell with issues relevant to our concerns over body composition, loss of abdominal visceral fat, and preservation of muscle. By eliminating these relatively recent additions to the human diet, such as wheat and ultraprocessed foods, you take a big first step to reverting back to a diet that is programmed into your genetic code and physiology.

Later in *SUPER Body*, when we dive into the nitty-gritty details of what to eat, we will borrow from the many lessons that the *Wheat Belly* experience taught us, but add new insights that amplify the shape and body composition benefits.

THE VEGETARIAN LION

If you were left to fend for yourself in a wild environment without processed foods, supermarkets, food delivery services, or credit cards, how and what would you eat? Most of us wouldn't know what to do, given how far we've strayed from our dietary roots.

If the style of eating programmed into your genetic code means that you were meant to hunt down animals to slaughter for your next meal, supplemented by the roots, berries, nuts, leaves, birds' eggs, fish, and shellfish you gathered from the surrounding terrain, then what is this thing called the modern diet? It is a (mis-)interpretation of diet, a corruption of the human dietary script written into your DNA. It is inconsistent with the style of eating that humans adhered to for the first few million years that our species and predecessors walked this planet.

Just as a catfish or turtle follows a specific dietary menu written into its genetic code, so it goes with humans. Imagine you witness a lion gore a wildebeest, then consume its intestines, heart, and lungs. You're disgusted, so you capture the lion, confine it in a cage and feed it kale and broccoli—what happens to the lion? It dies, of course, likely within weeks. You may not like it, you may find it repulsive, but the lion has a way of eating and surviving that is programmed into its genetic code, behavior, and physiology. Humans are no different.

Regaining your dietary footing is actually quite simple, provided you are able to forget nearly all that you've been told. While there is no need to grab a spear or ax, you will need to choose foods as close to their original form as possible. An egg, piece of salmon, or avocado would qualify, as would an apple, onion, or slice of beef. But nothing advertised on television, advocated by conventional dietary guidelines, or that comes with glitzy multicolored packaging fits into this return-to-our-dietary-roots program. And there is no such things as "healthy whole grains."

In some ways, we might be grateful for the mistakes made in diet and health over the past half century because this has showed us, in graphic detail, how *not* to conduct our lives. Follow the path of conventional wisdom and you are destined to fail. Just go shopping at your favorite big-box store and witness what has happened to our species: Never before has such a dietary catastrophe afflicted human health, shape, and body composition.

Let's therefore revisit what constitutes a basic, fundamental, and evolutionarily adaptive way of eating that looks nothing like what most modern people do in their day-to-day consumption.

EAT IT WHOLE

If we therefore adhere to a style of eating that echoes the lifestyle followed by our preagricultural ancestors, we must reject many modern notions of healthy eating. We reject the idea of limiting intake of fat, saturated fat, and cholesterol. Bacon, pork fat, and butter are back on the menu. We avoid most processed foods and completely banish all ultraprocessed foods. There will be no frozen pizzas made with white flour, high-fructose corn syrup–laden tomato sauce, processed cheese, sodium nitrite, maltodextrin, BHA, or BHT. Therefore, there will be no corn or potato chips, sodas, breakfast cereals, instant noodles, sandwich bread, or potato flakes in our kitchens. Avoiding such foods also means that we have minimized exposure to preservatives, mixing and emulsifying agents, food colorings, and other unhealthy additives.

We reject the idea of reducing calories to lose weight, so we eat to satiety whenever we desire, accepting that our appetite will be reduced due to the increased satiety of consuming unlimited fats and oils, the removal of gliadin-derived opioid peptide appetite stimulants, and (as I shall discuss later) the increase in the hormone oxytocin we will experience that turns off our interest in between-meal snacking.

We therefore choose whole foods whenever possible. We can recognize whole foods because they typically have no labels, are rarely advertised, and can be found primarily in the produce area, at the butcher counter, and in the dairy and egg refrigerators. We have no need of the aisles and aisles of chips, breakfast cereals, and breads. We may have to occasionally venture into those aisles to retrieve nuts, such as almonds, walnuts, or pecans, or to navigate those aisles for safe condiments, such as mustards, horseradish, and no-sugar-added ketchup. And, of course, nonfood items, such as laundry detergent, are in those inner aisles. But most of our shopping time should be spent in the areas where real, whole foods are made available.

This change causes some people to panic and ask, "What's left?!" Be assured, plenty is left. If we don't limit fat, we can enjoy a generous serving of butter on our green beans, as much extra-virgin olive oil as we desire in our salad dressings. We can buy fatty cuts of meat (a rib eye steak, for example) and eat the fat as well as the meat. We avoid lean ground beef or pork but choose full-fat. When we consume poultry or fish, make sure to eat the skin. If we include dairy products, choose full-fat cream and milk, never skim or reduced fat. Vegetables and fruit are readily obtainable whole, but we choose produce that is organic whenever possible, not coated in any waxes or other substances, but limit some that have been cultivated and hybridized for high sugar content.

There are times when we choose foods that have undergone minimal processing. For example, we resort to ground almonds and ground flaxseed to use as flours to make muffins and pizza crust. Although they are ground and thereby partially processed, they do not have preservatives, emulsifiers, colorings, flavorings, or other unhealthy additives. We might purchase a premade salsa made with chopped onions, tomatoes, and cilantro but, once again, with no added emulsifiers or mixing agents (avoiding, of course, the occasional brands that do add unwanted ingredients). We supplement with fish oil capsules and vitamin D to compensate for deficiencies, unable to consume as much fish as we might prefer because of mercury contamination, and because we fail to obtain sufficient sun exposure due to latitude, work habits, and the societal expectation that we wear clothing in public. Because most of us find unacceptable the notion of adding back to our diet tongue and stomach, we resort to processed collagen peptides and hyaluronic acid with no added ingredients—imperfect, perhaps, but better than not obtaining those nutrients at all. Overall, there is no food with umpteen additives in this lifestyle.

A general rule: If a food looks as if it was just picked off a tree, dug up from the ground, or sliced off the animal, it is likely whole. If it comes with an ingredient list as long as your arm or is served at a drive-thru window, it is not. There are indeed times when we resort to including foods that have undergone some level of processing—few of us want to make our own mustard or harvest and roast our own coffee beans. But in general, we minimize consumption of processed foods, concentrating our choices on foods that our friend from 50,000 BC would recognize as food.

THE OFFAL TRUTH

If you're not familiar with the term "offal," then maybe "sweetbreads," "variety meats," or "chitterlings" will ring a bell. If not, your great-grandmother was certainly familiar with them. She never received advice to cut saturated fat and cholesterol from her diet, but simply followed traditional patterns of eating and food preparation handed down over countless prior generations. A century ago, people regularly ate liver, tongue, intestinal casings for their sausages, tripe from sheep and cows' stomachs, and other organ meats without blinking an eye. After all, there was a lot of time, work, and money invested in raising livestock, such as a cow. Throwing away the organs would be unthinkable.

Among the consequences of leaving organ meats out of the modern diet is a dramatic reduction in the intake of collagen and hyaluronic acid, two important dietary factors that affect shape and body composition. Our hearts, tongues, skin, and intestines are rich in collagen. Our brains and skin are especially rich in hyaluronic acid. Neglect intake of collagen and abdominal girth expands, and we lose muscle while also accelerating deterioration of joints and aging of skin. Neglect intake of hyaluronic acid and our skin becomes drier and more wrinkled, we lack joint (synovial) lubrication, and we fail to obtain the dramatic effects this fiber (yes: an animal-sourced form of fiber, unique among most other fibers that are plant sourced) has on GI microbes, with influence over insulin resistance and inflammation and thereby body shape and composition. So you see that there's so much lost by turning up our noses at offal. Modern people often express disgust when it comes to organ meats, so slaughterhouses and meat manufacturers divert organs for use in pet food; butchers are bewildered should you have the temerity to request some pancreas or kidney. Besides the benefits from meat (i.e., muscle), collagen, and hyaluronic acid, organ meat is nutrient rich especially in B vitamins such as B_{12}, omega-3 fatty acids, and fat-soluble vitamins. Most organs are rich in fat, adding to satiety and reducing desire for carbs and sugars.

I sympathize with those who simply cannot embrace a return to organ meats. However, you can compromise by mixing ground liver into ground beef, or making liver pâté, eating the skin on poultry or fish, or just making a habit of obtaining real sausage in casing (i.e., intestines) to get you used to consuming heart, thymus, or tongue. If you're still easing your way out of the "avoid fat and cholesterol" bandwagon, there are ways to obtain most of the benefits by engaging in simple practices, such as adding collagen or hyaluronic acid powdered supplements to yogurts, kefirs, smoothies, or other familiar foods. Don't make the mistake of adopting bone broths, which have become a popular way to obtain such nutrients as collagen. Bone broths, home-made or commercial, have been shown to have high levels of the heavy metal lead (especially when vinegar is added to increase mineral release from bone, a practice that doubles lead levels in the broth).[17,18] Instead, follow the safer practice of making the admittedly unappetizing-sounding "carcass broth," broths and soups made from the remains of an animal—some bones included, no vinegar, boiled for shorter peri-ods of time, such as 3 or 4 hours, less than the 36 or so hours used to make bone broth. Include any leftover meat, organs, fats, skin, tendons, and ligaments, rich in the factors we are after: fats, collagen, and hyal-uronic acid.

THE END OF THE LOW-FAT ERA

It has been a blunder of breathtaking proportions, exported to most corners of the modern world: the message to reduce consumption of fat, saturated fat, and cholesterol.

The most shocking thing about this fifty-year social experiment is that there never was sufficient evidence to support such a shift in human dietary habits in the first place, certainly not what would pass for proof in our twenty-first-century understanding of credible human clinical trial evidence. Not long ago, heart disease was rare, and now it is a multibillion-dollar franchise for the health-care system.

The reduction in fat and cholesterol intake left a calorie gap that had to be filled to satisfy appetites. In other words, you cannot just reduce fat intake and not compensate to fill the lost calories, as most people will cave into hunger signals. When we reduce fat, the major-ity of people will increase carbohydrate and sugar intake. Sometimes, it takes the form of whole-grain bagels; sometimes, it's a bag of corn chips or quart of low-fat ice milk. When carb and sugar content of our diet is increased, insulin resistance increases, measures such as blood sugar and blood pressure increase, and abdominal fat expands.[19] When severe, as in abdominal obesity, ectopic fat accumulates, accelerating disease across multiple organs. Even muscle can become infiltrated by fat, reducing strength and erasing many of the health advantages of maintaining healthy muscle, a situation labeled as "myosteatosis," an especially unhealthy process that I shall discuss later in the book. And it is becoming clear that fatty infiltration of muscle has become an explosive problem, worsening with aging and common dietary habits.[20] Fat in the diet is natural and physiologic because our body is fully capable of processing it; fat created by consumption of sugars, ultraprocessed foods, and other modern factors is not, causing fat to be deposited in locations where it does not belong.

Where did such unnatural ideas come from? Why would a departure from the diet that humans followed for the preceding thousands of generations, a diet that almost never resulted in coronary heart disease and type 2 diabetes, become so deeply ingrained in modern dietary dogma? That may be a story for another day, but much of that misguided "wisdom" originated with a form of analysis called observational evidence—not human clinical trials, but making crude and largely unfounded observations on the dietary behaviors of everyday people.

If you were to participate in one of these studies, you may be asked, for instance, "What did you have for breakfast on Monday?" You answer, "I think I had some oatmeal with skim milk and a banana." "How about lunch?" You respond, "Well, I ate at my desk at work, so I had a ham sandwich with mayonnaise on rye with some cottage cheese." "What did you have for dinner?" You answer, "That was the night I had dinner at a local restaurant with my spouse and another couple, so I had a plate of spaghetti and meatballs, Italian bread with butter, and a green salad with Italian dressing, then two glasses of Chianti." Then, someone contacts you ten years later and asks whether you've had a heart attack, developed type 2 diabetes, or colon cancer. In the interval since you provided your diet survey responses, you've gained and lost weight three times, experienced a divorce accompanied by two years of extreme stress, your two children got married, and you had a parent and close friend pass away, diet habits seesawing wildly over the years. You had periods of binge drinking, periods of abstinence, a few months of going almost entirely to fast-food restaurants, a period when you engaged in a liver "cleanse"—drinking only lemon water and apple cider vinegar, a trip to Italy, a handful of vacations to the Caribbean as well as a cruise or two. In short, your food habits from ten years earlier do not even come close to reflecting what happened over the ensuing decade. Yet this laughable and completely unreliable method of generating a several-day dietary snapshot many years earlier is the basis for dietary guidelines and much dietary advice. This explains why media headlines one day read "Eggs cause heart disease" and then, a few months later, declare "Eggs unrelated to heart disease." Or "Red meats associated with colon cancer" followed by "Red meats unassociated with colon cancer." Such surveys of eating habits are not evidence. They are misleading momentary glimpses that do not reflect the enormous variation and unpredictability of human life over time.

This several decades–long dietary information misadventure has led to all the mantras of conventional dietary advice, all based on a dietary house of cards that topples with the slightest breeze. These awful dietary mistakes led modern people to abandon consumption of organ meats and adopt perverse and illogical practices, such as choosing skim milk over whole, throwing away bacon grease or avoiding bacon altogether, or buying boneless, skinless chicken breast absent some of the most important ingredients of all.

As bad as the modern diet situation has become, it gets worse.

"DID YOU WANT FRIES WITH THAT?"

To make money in the food industry, the equation is simple: Provide products with the lowest production costs possible, then sell to consumers for as high a price as the market will bear. It often means cutting corners on quality of ingredients, resorting to low-cost fillers, such as cornstarch, wheat flour, and sugar; extending shelf life as much as possible with preservatives; adding emulsifying agents to keep the food looking aesthetically pleasing; and taking advantage of ingredients that amplify appetite. And finally, wrapping the whole thing in eye-catching packaging, adding a cartoon character or sports figure, or even an endorsement from the American Heart Association or other agency, then tempting consumers with clever marketing.

What gets lost in this highly processed mix are vitamins, minerals, micronutrients, polyphenols, and other phytonutrients. One dietary casualty that stands out with relevance to our concerns for shape and body composition: carotenoids.

Carotenoids are the orange, red, and yellow pigments occurring in such foods as red and yellow peppers, carrots, and squash. There's beta-carotene, for instance, rich in carrots and egg yolks, and lycopene from tomatoes. Lutein and zeaxanthin, biochemical mirror images of each other, are sourced from these same foods, as well as from green leafy vegetables, such as kale and spinach. Astaxanthin is an orange-colored carotenoid naturally occurring in salmon, shrimp, trout, and shellfish, as well as produced by bacteria, algae, and some plants in small quantities. A 6-ounce serving of wild-caught salmon, for example, provides around 4 milligrams of astaxanthin. If compared to other carotenoids in antioxidant capacity, astaxanthin is tenfold more potent.[21]

Humans are unable to synthesize the hundreds of different carotenoids we require, and therefore we must rely entirely on dietary intake. If you were to set out today to harvest wild plants from the forest or jungle, you would obtain substantial quantities of carotenoids. In contrast, the carotenoid content of many modern popular foods is low or negligible. The shift away from crude plant matter to highly processed foods has caused carotenoid intake in Americans to plummet to low levels.[21,22]

Astaxanthin shines in minimizing inflammation, which provides benefits for eye health, diabetes, and coronary heart disease, but also in the reduction of abdominal visceral fat. Evidence suggests that a number of carotenoids have positive effects in reducing body fat, which you can obtain by the inclusion of the carotenoid-rich foods mentioned. But astaxanthin stands apart from other carotenoids as being the most potent regulator of metabolic factors and abdominal fat, likely via its capacity to reduce inflammation. Even by itself, astaxanthin has been shown, in human clinical studies, to reduce abdominal fat and waist circumference significantly.[23,24] Of course, the approach we take here will include astaxanthin, but we combine it with other factors that synergize and thereby amplify the body shape–modifying effects.

Modern aversion to carotenoid-rich foods, such as carrots, spinach, turnip greens, dandelion greens, and squash, has denied us the many health benefits of dietary carotenoids. Interestingly, low blood levels of carotenoids have an inverse relationship with obesity; that is, the more obese someone is, the lower their blood level of various carotenoids. Blood levels of carotenoids may therefore serve as an index of the quality of diet; the majority of people have painfully low levels.[25]

In the next chapter, let's consider in greater detail why such ideas as reducing calorie intake, achieved with a variety of different strategies, guarantees your failure and does not achieve long-term success, certainly not restoring control over determining which body distortions are where.

3

CALORIES IN, CALORIES OUT, AND OTHER FAIRY TALES

A S A CHILD, YOU MAY HAVE ENJOYED THE STORIES OF HANSEL and Gretel or Rip Van Winkle. But I doubt that you've drawn your life's lessons from such tales. You are not fooled by talk of evil witches kidnapping children or someone napping for twenty years. And yet most of the world clings to one fairy tale: that of cutting calories to lose weight.

At first blush, it makes sense: Reduce calorie intake while continuing to burn calories, and fat should melt off—if your body were a machine. But it's not. It is a well-designed, adaptive vessel that, above all else, will ensure survival should a reduction in food availability develop. If you and your clan returned from a hunt with little to show, or drought, wildfires, scavenging animals, or other factors caused foods you usually gathered to be in short supply and you and your family suffered the desperate gnaw of hunger, your body would work to ensure survival by reducing the rate at which it "burns" calories; that is, it will reduce your basal metabolic rate (BMR). This natural physiologic adaptation increased the likelihood that our ancestors would survive to see another sunrise, find a mate, raise children. Reduce calorie intake in our modern world, however, and your body cannot distinguish your weight-loss effort from starvation in the wild.

It is the dirty little secret of weight-loss programs: using pharmaceuticals to lose weight and having bariatric procedures that all rely on reducing calorie intake. Why ruin the party by telling you that study after study has demonstrated that, by reducing calories, you will initially lose weight, but the odds are overwhelming that you will regain it over time because of the drop in BMR?[1] You may have paid thousands of dollars and been given promises of fantastic weight-loss successes. Such approaches to losing weight can indeed result in losing 30, 50, or 100 pounds or more—at first. But basic human physiology kicks in and guarantees that the weight comes back, most of it within the first year after weight loss, regardless of how much money you paid or how much pain you endured in the process. This happens even if you maintain a low-calorie intake and exercise program.

Reduced-calorie diet strategies can take on a wide variety of shapes and sizes. In addition to the mantras repeated by doctors and dietitians, it could be a spouse shaming you into not reaching for seconds or batting down your hand as you reach for a bowl of Rocky Road ice cream. Some programs provide lists of "green, yellow, and red" foods, or a point system with higher points corresponding to higher-calorie foods, or smartphone-delivered admonishments to discourage you from giving into stress eating. It could even be a program that purports to individualize diet, specially created just for you to suit your physiology. But they are all variations on the same theme: reducing calorie intake.

Cutting calories has a long history of failure, with programs taking on incredibly varied and sometimes bizarre practices. Consuming a mixture of chamomile soap and vinegar, eating only Communion wafers, eating and purging, laxatives—there has been an endless list of useless calorie-restricting efforts employed by humans eager to lose weight.

Danalynne, 59

"In the '90s, Weight Watchers was 'the thing to do.' For me, each time I rejoined, I'd walk in and it was like a scene out of *Cheers*—instead of 'Norm,' it was 'Dana'! I was embarrassed as everyone knew my name and probably was known as the group flunky chunky girl. My belief, [as for] many, was that the number on the scale defined me. The lower the number, the better I was.

"Weighing in the mid-200s at that time, I was allotted more points than most. I would nosh on celery, carrots, and ranch dressing during the day, salted and roasted soybeans for that before dinner snack (you know, the one to stave off a bad dinner). I had 20 some points left and so 8–12 oz. of pasta with Romano cheese was what made this girl very happy. I adhered to the points, watched my sodium intake, did Richard Simmons's routines, only to be ridiculed at weigh-in as I lost only 4 ounces. I was even told that I couldn't have been doing things correctly because, at my weight, I should have lost at least 5 lbs.

"I lost more than weight: money, time, and self-esteem. I gained back the 20 lbs over the five-year on/off relationship with WW plus another 15 lbs. I never want to hear about WW again. Learning to like myself after many years of hatred."

CUTTING CALORIES: A LONG AND INGLORIOUS HISTORY

I've discussed how and why reducing calorie intake, regardless of method, no matter how enticing the sales pitch, will rarely yield long-term success in losing weight and managing body contours. But, because reduced calorie intake does indeed yield short-term weight loss, this cockroach of dietary advice refuses to die, surviving even the nuclear holocaust of scientific evidence to the contrary. So let's explore a bit further why this fiction of weight loss continues despite overwhelming evidence to the contrary.

Although the magnitude of overweight and obesity in times past was nowhere near crisis levels as it is in our times, prior populations, especially among the aristocracy, employed their versions of cutting calorie intake. Ancient Greeks had their version of reduced-calorie intake, as did the Romans and every other civilization since humans first congregated in villages and cities, entertaining all manner of fictions to engage this practice. Not unlike "treatments" used to manage syphilis, insanity, or homosexuality, these methods were often bizarre, sometimes dangerous or fatal. Forced vomiting and enemas were perennial favorites, as was fasting, often for prolonged periods.

Even over the last century or two, efforts to limit calorie intake have taken on a number of extreme forms, reflecting the desperation with which people pursue their weight-loss goals. During the Victorian era, women constricted their waists with corsets to discourage intake of food by physically compressing the stomach. In the early twentieth century, San Francisco businessman Horace Fletcher received wide popularity for advocating chewing each mouthful of food up to one hundred times—"Fletcherizing"—until solid food was liquefied, a strategy he boasted reduced calorie intake. The "Tapeworm Diet" was briefly popular, in which a capsule containing a live tapeworm was swallowed so that it took up residence in the gastrointestinal tract and consumed calories. Of course, people also became ill, sometimes seriously.[2]

It also wasn't uncommon over the years to use shame to coerce people into reducing calorie intake, equating obesity, for instance, with moral corruption. Despite the uselessness of such maneuvers, doctors to this day remain notorious for criticizing people for their weight, expressing disgust for their patients' lack of willpower or submitting to gluttony, blaming the patient for their weight struggles. We now know that "fat shaming" is counterproductive, as it worsens an already low sense of self-esteem, increases the likelihood of depression and feelings of helplessness, and may even result in the opposite: weight gain.[3] And then, of course, if asked how to accomplish weight loss, the doctor tells patients to "move more, eat less" or some other version of ineffective advice that nearly always backfires.

To this day, the fiction of reducing calories by whatever means dominates dietary thinking. We may no longer embrace such outdated and ineffective methods as excessive chewing or implanting intestinal parasites, but the same old worn and ineffective advice to reduce calorie intake persists.

If you are trying to lose weight, you are not alone. In any single year, about half the US population is trying to shed pounds by one means or another.[4] The appetite for the newest or shiniest program is therefore insatiable, fueling growth of a $150 billion per year industry. And the newest and shiniest will invariably involve some form of calorie restriction. Novelty takes on many forms: a new celebrity endorsement, a smartphone app that promises exciting new ways to avoid foods, ways to time your eating habits, shifting the order in which you consume foods, the newest GLP-1 agonist weight-loss drug.

Pharmaceuticals reduce food intake by blocking appetite hormones and creating nausea, resulting in loss of interest in food. The macaroni and cheese or strawberry cheesecake that previously made your mouth water no longer holds your interest. A procedure to place a constricting band around your stomach reduces the volume of the stomach, causing you to be satiated with less food: caloric restriction. Gastric bypass, in which the small intestine is rerouted to the upper portion of the stomach, reducing stomach volume to a small pouch, is no different. No matter how fancy or how costly or how enthusiastically they are promoted, these are *all* forms of calorie restriction. And we now know, with good evidence, that restricting calories, regardless of the form it takes, can indeed yield short-term weight loss but guarantees long-term regain of the weight.

Let's face it: Anyone who has purposefully and consciously reduced calorie intake knows that it is absolute misery. Deny yourself food and you will experience an overwhelming desire to eat, enviously eyeing other people's food, obsessing over when your next meal will come, even if it only consists of celery and cottage cheese. The availability of weight-loss drugs and bariatric procedures may therefore represent an improvement over just reducing calorie intake, as they remove the desperation and hunger component of reducing calories. Weight-loss drugs can make you indifferent to food, causing you to forget just how wonderful a slice of chocolate cheesecake felt on the tongue. Or the gastric bypass or lap-band made you feel full after just two bites of lasagna. Minus the misery, these two popular ways of reducing calorie intake are therefore offered as improvements over just pushing the plate away. In reality, they are incremental improvements that do not circumvent the problems associated with cutting calories; they just make it less miserable.

It's therefore all the same in the end: You regain the weight and you will once again be in the market for another program, drug, or procedure to lose the weight. For people and companies who make money from the weight-loss industry, it's the gift that keeps on giving. Sign up for yet another diet program, another prescription, lay out another several hundred to thousands of dollars to engage in another variation on cutting calories. It is not uncommon for someone to engage in dozens of programs over a lifetime, nearly always regaining most or all of the weight with each effort.

There is nothing magical about any of these approaches as *they are all the same*, just with varied outward appearances, different labels that fool the unsuspecting consumer. Incredibly, when the long-term failures of these programs become evident, it causes many—including doctors—to blame the individual and urge them to cut calories even more. The entire collection of blunders is encapsulated by the statement often attributed to Albert Einstein: "Insanity is doing the same thing over and over and expecting different results." It's useless: The strategy of reducing calories to lose weight essentially guarantees failure.

The long-term rebound of weight is therefore due to a basic survival mechanism that applies to all creatures, great and small: Reduce calorie intake and the body perceives deprivation or starvation. Your body cannot distinguish reduced calorie intake that results from a pharmaceutical or bariatric procedure from failing to kill an animal in the wild or failure to harvest sufficient roots and plants because of drought or cold weather. You may have paid plenty of money for the gastric bypass or weight-loss drug, but your body is indifferent to which method of weight loss you chose—it still thinks that you are at risk for dying of starvation. Your body therefore ratchets down the rate at which your body "burns" calories, to keep you from dying; that is, it reduces your BMR. Without this fail-safe mechanism, you would succumb to a basic fact of life on this planet: Lack of food means that you may be approaching death from starvation. Death from starvation occurs all the time, every day, around the world. The physiologic response of reduced BMR in the face of reduced food intake is therefore a "cushion," your body's built-in, genetically programmed safety measure to keep you alive.

WEIGHT LOSS IS NOT JUST FAT LOSS

Problem: All conventional methods of weight loss that involve reducing calorie intake will lead to loss of muscle.[5] Your biceps and triceps will be smaller, chest and back muscles deflated, thigh and calf muscles reduced in volume and strength. Loss of muscle will also involve the face and neck, often yielding the gaunt and wrinkled look that lost muscle can confer, not uncommonly giving you the appearance of having aged ten or more years. It's the source of an incredible amount of frustration for people trying to lose weight and keep it off: Can't we just lose fat and not muscle? Muscle, after all, helps you walk, climb, fight, and navigate the world, not fat.

Muscle mass is the primary determinant of BMR. Think of BMR as the rate at which your body metabolizes calories all day, every day for the work of living. Even if a reduced-calorie lifestyle is maintained following weight loss, weight will be regained due to the drop in BMR. Deny yourself second helpings, or turn away the butter on your scrambled eggs or steak, and you have unknowingly planted a trap for yourself that will catch you a few months later, causing you to regain the weight you worked so hard to lose.

Reduced calorie intake, regardless of how it is achieved, therefore leads to weight loss that is 25 percent lost muscle, sometimes more. You can easily regain fat, but you regain almost none of the muscle you've lost. In addition to taking away control over BMR and weight, losing that much muscle also poses long-term risk that will impair your ability to navigate your environment, like weakness in climbing stairs or carrying groceries, hormonal disruptions, increased susceptibility to such conditions as dementia and heart disease, frailty, falls, and fractures.[6] Loss of muscle during weight loss is not benign, and it compounds the 30 percent loss of muscle that develops simply due to the aging process. Control over our weight therefore becomes harder and harder as we age, largely due to the age-related loss of muscle and reduced BMR, worsened by conventional efforts to lose weight.

Lonnie and Carrie

"ONE YEAR AGO TODAY, MY LIFE CHANGED IN UNTHINKABLE ways. I discovered the *Wheat Belly 10-Day Grain Detox* book and read it during my kids' spring break. I had dabbled in the 'Paleo' diet world a bit over the last five years with inconsistent success and had some idea about how good I felt when eliminating grains.

"But the protocols in this book seemed to go further than just diet, like addressing vitamin, nutrient, hormone, and gut flora deficiencies from living our modern lifestyles and eating the 'civilized' diet. I knew deep down that I needed to try this detox for 10 days, and asked my wife to begin this journey with me.

"We decided to start on a Friday so that we had the weekend to deal with the detox symptoms (which honestly was not that difficult for us). We made it through the first 5 days, and by day 6 I felt like a completely different person. Better sleep, much more energy, and an almost euphoric feeling that I cannot describe. This feeling continued for days, then weeks, then months. The weight poured off us with little physical effort (over 80 lbs between us, 40+ each). Brain fog was gone. Aches and pains disappeared. Food tasted better. We received countless compliments about how much younger we looked."

Reaccumulation of fat without return of muscle worsens the processes of insulin resistance and inflammation, not only making it tougher to lose weight again in future and compounding age-related changes but also tipping the scales in favor of developing serious health problems.[7] Engage in this cycle of weight loss and weight regain repeatedly—"yo-yo dieting" or "weight cycling"—and you can appreciate that permanent weight loss becomes increasingly out of reach, even impossible, while also adding to health struggles.

People invest not only money but plenty of emotional currency in the hopes of once again fitting into the beloved pair of jeans from ten or twenty years ago or a dress size in the single digits. It is not just disappointing to have the lost weight return, it is also demoralizing and embarrassing. It's a good thing you didn't discard the clothes in your plus-size wardrobe because, by engaging in conventional efforts, you're going to need them again. It doesn't help that the people around you continue to point fingers, believing some moral or behavioral weakness is responsible. Understand this crucial fact: It is *not* a result of weakness and it is *not* your fault. It is a result of fatally flawed dietary thinking and failure to recognize the importance of body composition.

THE WEIGHT-LOSS IED

The Biggest Loser TV show, airing for nearly twenty years, puts on display an extreme version of "move more, eat less." Overweight participants are put on a reduced-calorie diet (about 50% of usual calorie intake) and three or more hours per day of exercise, both aerobic and resistance training. Losing 10 pounds per week, sometimes 20 pounds, is common, accompanied by plenty of sobbing and emotional breakdowns due to the rigors of the program, but participants are bolstered by hopes of winning the $250,000 prize for the most weight lost.

Graduates of the eighth season of the TV show were studied by researchers at the National Institutes of Health (NIH). Their assessment revealed that, despite the extraordinary amounts of weight lost, nearly all participants regained the weight after leaving the show—

despite maintaining a low-calorie diet and exercise program. The NIH scientific group measured BMR among show participants after graduating the program. Their measurements revealed that graduates experienced a 27 percent reduction in BMR that persisted for the six-year duration of the study.[8] (Because the study ended after six years, it is likely that the reduced BMR persisted for even longer—it is, for practical purposes, permanent or nearly permanent.) In short, reduced calories, and thereby reduced BMR, virtually guaranteed regain of weight, even if a low-calorie intake and exercise program were maintained, and this effect persisted for many years. The intensive exercise program that included strength exercises reduced muscle loss from the usual 25 percent of lost weight to 19 percent, but even these heroic efforts did not block regain of fat weight. Despite the loss of substantial amounts of weight, despite the emotionally turbulent process, despite the intense coaching and diet supervision, weight regain was assured due to the loss of muscle and resultant drop in BMR. The study documented that regain of weight was due not to overindulgence, nor to sloth, but to a biological survival response. The researchers stated that "Weight loss is accompanied by a slowing of resting metabolic rate that is often greater than would be expected based on the measured changes in body composition. This phenomenon is called 'metabolic adaptation' or 'adaptive thermogenesis' and acts to counter weight loss and is thought to contribute to weight regain."[8]

Weight lost by calorie reduction, regardless of method, on- or off-camera, regardless of the agony endured, *ensures* weight regain in the majority. And the regained weight is mostly fat, not muscle, meaning that, despite the extreme effort and discipline, body shape and composition deteriorate further. The reduction in metabolic rate that persists for many years after such efforts makes future weight-loss efforts even more difficult or impossible.

Proponents of the idea of "a calorie is a calorie"—for example, 100 calories of sugar is the same as 100 calories of olive oil—argue that it is consistent with the laws of thermodynamics: The energy entering a system must equal the energy leaving a system. It allows arguments that overweight and obesity are products of overeating and inactivity:

Energy enters the system (your body), and energy either leaves the system through activity or is stored as fat. In this line of thinking, the energy entering must equal the energy leaving or stored. This overly simplistic thinking has dominated dietary advice for many years. But the laws of thermodynamics fail to factor in the spectacular differences in the living human body: different levels of insulin that determine whether fat is gained or lost, differing hormonal status, different gastrointestinal microbiomes (the composition of microbes in the gut that take nutrients and convert them to various metabolites), many of which influence weight. Viewing all calories as equal also ignores differences in foods, such qualities as caloric density, fiber content, and nutrient accessibility. If a calorie is a calorie, there would be no difference between the 2,000 calories of a quart of strawberry ice cream and the 2,000 calories in 38 cups of fresh strawberries. (The strawberry ice cream, for instance, likely contains polysorbate 80, carboxymethylcellulose, and carrageenan to discourage separation, factors that add to long-term increased abdominal fat accumulation by impairing the intestinal mucus barrier.[9]) In other words, your body is not a wax-burning candle or an electric motor; it is a complex biological machine with numerous factors that vary how a calorie is handled, with different inputs (calories, fat, protein, carbohydrates, fibers) yielding different end effects.

Cutting calories also increases the release of hormones that amplify the intensity of hunger, hormones such as ghrelin, glucose-dependent insulinotropic polypeptide, and pancreatic polypeptide. Cutting calories also reduces hormones, such as cholecystokinin and amylin, that "turn off" appetite. These are changes that develop as you cut calories to lose weight but that also persist *even after all the weight is regained*, leaving you hungrier and less able to control eating behavior.[10,11] With reduced BMR and perverse distortions of hormones that drive hunger, it is *harder to control weight after weight loss*. This phenomenon persists even after fat weight is regained and is, for all practical purposes, permanent, or at least long-lasting. Cutting calories is misery to begin with. After losing, then regaining, weight, it is even more miserable, all part of your body's normal and natural response to protect you from starvation and death.

DANNY CAHILL'S *BIGGEST LOSER* EXPERIENCE

Danny Cahill's *Biggest Loser* weight-loss success at age 40 was nothing short of meteoric. Starting at a weight of 430 pounds, he lost an astounding 239 pounds over two hundred days of his participation in the popular TV show, 24 pounds in the first week alone, a testimony to this man's emotional strength and commitment. The extraordinary weight-loss success earned him the winning spot on season 8 and prize money for his efforts. Jillian Michaels, one of the show's coaches, told him that the 800 calories-per-day diet he followed was the most severe of any male participant ever in the history of the show. Despite the extreme calorie deprivation that resulted from this starvation level of food intake, coupled with many hours per day of resistance and aerobic exercise, estimated to require around 8,000 calories per day, he stayed the course over the seven months. At his final weigh-in, show hostess Alison Sweeney declared, "Because it's not just about changing your body, it's about transforming your life."

From what you now know, Danny's incredible initial success was inevitably destined to be followed by a return to his prior weight and health struggles.

In my interview with Danny, who was very gracious in sharing his story, he related that, in the hopes of not regaining the weight, he maintained a two-or-more-hours-per-day exercise schedule, six days per week, along with a severely reduced-calorie lifestyle after leaving the show. "I would go back to reunions and I would see people, other contestants that were on seasons before me, regaining the weight. I was the 'Biggest Loser' at the time, broke every record. But I didn't understand what was going to happen after the show. My metabolism had slowed down, but my hunger increased." Sadly, despite his heroic efforts, he has regained nearly all the weight.

Danny was also one of the fourteen participants studied after season 8 by NIH scientists after their weight-loss experience, with all but one regaining all the weight. Like the others who regained weight, Danny also showed the dramatic reduction in metabolic rate that resulted—and persisted—for long after the show ended.

A number of human clinical studies in which various "isocaloric" (same number of calories) diets were compared reveal distinct differences in outcomes. For example, diets that reduce carbohydrates time and again have proven superior to diets that limit fats, yielding greater reductions in weight, body fat, and waist circumference when carbs are limited.[12] Despite this up-front advantage, even diets that limit carbohydrate intake, just as with limiting calories, also lead to loss of muscle and thereby weight regain for the majority. Low-carb diets in their various forms thereby represent an improvement over simple reduction of calories or fat, but we can still do better.

Despite the billions of dollars spent every year on such programs, despite hype and marketing, programs that reduce calories, regardless of how this is achieved, have been a huge failure. Whether corsets to compress stomach volume, a pharmaceutical that induces nausea and indifference to food, or a doctor shaming you into eating more lettuce and fewer tortilla chips, long-term success will be unattainable. Despite the proven deficiencies of calorie-reduced approaches, billions of dollars continue to be spent every year on bariatric procedures, GLP-1 pharmaceutical agents, and weight-loss programs, all enjoying vigorous growth.

Reducing calories is a fool's errand. It may make entertaining TV, but it is ruinous for management of weight, body composition, health, and self-esteem. And, ironically, the people with the greatest success in initially losing the most weight—the biggest loser—are also the people who gain back the most weight.

In Part 2, let's consider why maintenance of muscle during weight loss is a critical factor and why this is the key to restoring youthful shape and body composition. You can't increase muscle by cutting calories, you can't increase muscle with a GLP-1 agonist or other drug, and you can't increase muscle by undergoing a bariatric procedure. Including a vigorous resistance training can only partially blunt the loss but not prevent it. Preserving or increasing muscle requires some unique and unexpected strategies that are safe, effective, and inexpensive, and yield a long list of other health benefits. I can assure you: There will be no calorie counting, no reducing fat intake, no extreme exercise, no hours spent at the gym hefting barbells or dumbbells, and no assigning personal blame.

PART II

THE GUT-MUSCLE AXIS

I T'S A REVOLUTIONARY CONCEPT: THE TRILLIONS OF MICRO-scopic creatures living in the 30 feet of your gastrointestinal (GI) tract are in open communication with the rest of your body. They "talk" to your brain, skin, thyroid gland, breasts, uterus, urinary bladder, and, yes, to the muscles of your body. They also communicate with the various depots of fat. And those body parts also "talk" back to microbes, influencing their behavior. Unfortunately, this wonderful system of "cross talk" has gone haywire in modern people, posing implications for numerous health conditions from the brain on down, including determining where and how much fat is deposited and how much muscle you maintain.

We are going to do something wonderful and powerful to give you back control over this phenomenon: We are going to give you tools that allow your GI microbes to communicate with muscle and fat, microbes that influence the location and quantity of abdominal fat, restore musculature to the state you enjoyed many years earlier, increase metabolic rate, as well as provide more youthful skin, improve mental health, provide benefits for reproductive health, amplify immune response, and even improve your social life.

And there's what I call the "loudspeaker effect": Benefits obtained through changes in diet, restoration of nutrients lacking in modern life, and other positive efforts are all amplified when we pay attention to our microbiomes. Life and health are better when we intelligently enlist the assistance of the trillions of microbes that can be at our beck and call, provided you know how to speak their "language." Let this section of SUPER Body be the start of a very interesting conversation.

4

MUSCLE YOUR WAY TO YOUTHFUL SHAPE AND BODY COMPOSITION

WELL-PLACED LUMPS, BUMPS, AND BULGES ARE AN ADVANTAGE. They make you more attractive, healthier, and more youthful, with the redistribution of fat and muscle also yielding metabolic advantage. Read a marketing pitch for a weight-loss program, however, or the warnings of side effects from a weight-loss drug, or receive the urgings of your doctor to undergo a bariatric procedure, and you will not encounter any mention of the inevitable loss of muscle.

Unfortunately, some people are turned off by discussions of muscle. A bodybuilder's physique isn't universally attractive. Don't worry: No one here is going to develop 21-inch biceps or deep pectoral grooves, massive muscle that requires hours and hours at the gym. The muscle I am talking about here refers to regaining muscle you've lost through the process of aging, with added, often dramatic, muscle loss that resulted from losing weight by reducing calories. We therefore beat back the effects of aging and atrophy, as well as undoing the effects of previous dietary mistakes. Men, having greater muscle mass than women, will gain a bit more with these strategies, but the return of youthful muscle cuts across both sex and age.

So, in this chapter, we'll focus on the critical importance of muscle. You won't be wowing friends with your big biceps or heavily muscled thighs bursting the seams on your shorts, but you can restore youthful muscle that you enjoyed, coupled with all its metabolic benefits, in your twenties. You can indeed push the bar further and add additional muscle by, say, incorporating some push-ups or a few minutes with resistance machines or weights, but it is not necessary. Instead, we are going to reverse the factors that allowed you to lose youthful muscle and thereby regain the advantages of youthful physiology. Even if you are reading this as a young person, know that, despite your youth, you also lack multiple factors that affect shape and body composition, the loss of which will eventually catch up with you. And you, like the rest of us, are exposed to factors that will lead to bulging abdomens, expansive buttocks, and impaired musculature.

It is a reality of life: We lose muscle and strength as we age. Most people reach their peak level of muscle mass around the age of twenty-five to thirty years, the greatest lifelong quantity of muscle in their faces, chests, necks, backs, thighs, and elsewhere, as well as the greatest level of strength. After that age, we experience a steady decline. The process of aging typically involves loss of 30–35 percent of muscle from our peak.[1] People who engage in strenuous physical exercise involving resistance—for instance, weight lifting, track events, or speed skating, among other activities—may decline more slowly due to their training efforts, but they will nonetheless also experience muscle loss with aging. Others who engage in strenuous labor, such as laying brick, roofing, or other efforts involving heavy lifting, can likewise maintain muscle longer than others, but they, too, will experience age-related decline. Speaking generally, however, especially applying to those of us whose maximum physical effort may be pushing around a computer mouse or chopping onions, we all lose significant amounts of muscle as we age.

Dan, 52

"WHAT SETS THIS CHAPTER OF MY LIFE APART IS THE SUS-
tainability of my weight loss over the past two years, coupled
with continued improvements in my physical fitness. Surprisingly, I no longer experience food cravings, an astonishing change that I attribute to a better understanding of the
gut microbiome.

"The transformation has been remarkable. Not only have
I maintained my weight loss, but my relationship with food
has fundamentally changed. The once irresistible urges for
certain foods have vanished, allowing me to make more
conscious choices about my nutrition. This shift in my diet,
along with my commitment to physical activity, has been
instrumental in sustaining my health gains."

You can clearly see the loss of muscle in someone unburdened by
excess fat: skinny arms and legs, deflated pectoral and back muscles,
flaccid facial features marked by deep wrinkles and jowls. Of course,
if buried under subcutaneous fat (fat just below the skin surface), it
may partially conceal the loss of muscle, but atrophied muscle is there
nonetheless. The net loss of muscle mass can be staggering. It means
that, the older we get, the more muscle we lose, the lower our BMR,
and we thereby retain less and less control over weight, shape, and
body composition and can gain significant fat weight even with a low
calorie intake.

Most of us don't even think about muscle during an effort to
lose weight. If you've attempted calorie-restrictive weight loss, you
were probably more focused on a number on a scale or the circumference of your waist than you were on your muscles. The amount
of muscle you have can make or break a weight-loss effort, as well as
exert major influence on the location of your bulges, good and bad.
There is even evidence that loss of muscle affects mortality; that is, it

can shorten your life.[2] Loss of muscle is therefore pivotal, determining how you look, your susceptibility to modern diseases, your ability to control weight and fat distribution, and even your life span.[3]

RESISTANCE TRAINING: A WASTED EFFORT?

It is clear that losing muscle during any weight-loss effort therefore plants a ticking time bomb that ensures regain of weight. Can efforts to preserve muscle mass during weight loss block this phenomenon? Can, for instance, an intensive resistance training program during weight loss preserve muscle and avoid the downturn in BMR? When I discuss this issue with colleagues, they assure me that, provided someone engages in resistance training during their GLP-1 injections, for instance, muscle loss with weight-loss efforts will not be a problem. Is this true?

No, it is not true. Muscle building via strength or resistance training can modestly blunt the effect but cannot block it entirely. Refer back to the NIH study of *The Biggest Loser* participants: three or more hours per day of exercise that included rigorous resistance training, efforts that blunted but did not prevent loss of muscle, yet all the weight was regained.[3] Another NIH study involved obese participants who reduced calorie intake by 30 percent and engaged in two hours per day of resistance and aerobic exercise six days per week—an extraordinary twelve hours per week of exercise. Participants lost an impressive amount of weight over thirty weeks: an average of 126.7 pounds, of which 23.1 pounds was muscle, representing 18 percent of the weight lost, less than the usual 25 percent that occurs without resistance training, but not enough to fully block muscle loss and the BMR-reducing effect it brings.[4] Participants' BMR was formally measured and found to have plunged by a breathtaking 789 calories per day (i.e., their bodies "burned" that much fewer calories per day). It means that, even if you restricted daily calorie intake to an agonizing 1,200 calories per day, you will still regain fat weight. Just as with *The Biggest Loser* participants, the drop in BMR means that, even if a low-calorie diet and exercise program are maintained, weight regain is unstoppable. And reduced BMR persists for many years after the initial weight loss coupled, of course, with the distortions in appetite hormones that leave you hungrier even after you regain the weight—talk about getting kicked after you fall down.

Another interesting phenomenon was observed in one of the NIH studies: Weight loss was paralleled by a 44 percent reduction in the T3 thyroid hormone.[4] The T3 hormone is the main active form of thyroid hormone responsible for metabolic rate. In this low-T3 situation, people complain of becoming fatigued more easily, sleeping excessively, losing hair, and experiencing dry skin, constipation, and weight gain. T3 is therefore a major determinant of metabolic rate that drops with the inevitable loss of muscle during a weight-loss effort. It is the body's response when presented with what is perceived as starvation and a threat to survival. In other words, as noble and effort intensive as such programs can be, the body's survival instincts kick in, including changes in hormonal levels that block your weight-loss ambitions. Your body's normal and natural physiologic response will work against your weight-loss efforts to keep you alive. (And, by the way, this is a phenomenon that is foreign or unrecognized by most practicing physicians who rarely look beyond a thyroid-stimulating hormone [TSH] level to assess thyroid status. It specifically requires measurement of "free T3"; i.e., the T3 thyroid hormone not bound by proteins but free to exert beneficial effects.)

Efforts that involve resistance training to preserve muscle therefore can only partially blunt the loss of muscle. Loss of muscle ignites a basic survival mechanism that no calorie counting, smartphone app, amount of chewing, or daily trips to the gym can circumvent. You can therefore begin to appreciate that the pivotal issue that dictates whether long-term weight-loss success is achieved is *muscle*: You absolutely must not lose muscle during an effort to lose weight. If you do, BMR drops, your T3 thyroid hormone level drops, and weight regain is assured. You will experience greater hunger and may even shave several years off your life span. In *SUPER Body*, one of our priorities is to therefore preserve or increase muscle and not permit its loss to booby-trap your future ability to achieve your desired goals.

As we shall discuss, it is possible to maintain muscle at—or even increase it back to—youthful levels and thereby not lose the advantages of higher BMR. We can also specifically target abdominal visceral fat that is the driver of insulin resistance and inflammation, which will further reshape body composition. We will take lessons from emerging science that draw advantages from some unexpected places. These shape- and body composition–molding practices will involve restoring gastrointestinal microbes that modern people have lost, restoring body-shaping hormones, such as oxytocin; reducing body-distorting hormones, such as cortisol; and correcting the many dietary mistakes that most of us have made because we were led to believe that dietary guidelines were crafted from good science. Taken all together, this is a formula for restoring youthful body shape and composition that is virtually effortless, does not involve hunger or reduction in calories, and rejects most modern notions of weight loss and healthy eating.

Simply stated, much of the advantage gained by these unconventional methods revolves around preservation or increase in muscle. Muscle is our friend: The more muscle you have, the greater your metabolic rate and therefore the more you are in control over weight gain or loss. Healthy youthful musculature (again: not to be confused with the steroid-laden, bloated muscularity of the bodybuilding world) also has long-term health benefits, such as protection from falls, injury, fractures, frailty, and loss of independence. More muscle also protects us from loss of bone density while also maintaining testosterone levels in males and preserving healthy flexibility and mobility in everyone.

REBUILDING LOST MUSCLE

Preserving or increasing muscle will not require grueling hours lifting weights at the gym. A modest effort at resistance training can improve your results, but it is not necessary. You can indeed gain several pounds of muscle as this is the phenomenon that restores control over loss of fat—it's not a detriment, but an advantage. You may notice that your shoulders and arms are firmer, thighs and calves regain the restored musculature of youth, climbing stairs or riding a bike up hills becomes easier. Even facial features can become more youthful with a smoother forehead, less prominent crow's-feet and worry lines, less saggy neck-lines, all due to restoration of youthful muscle. So get over it: If you witness an increase in weight in the early part of your *SUPER Body* program, I urge you to recognize this as a *good* thing, as it means that you are regaining muscle and thereby control over your BMR and the ability to reshape body contours.

We are going to restore lost muscle by drawing from some unique strategies that involve participating in the "conversation" between gut microbes and muscle, a conversation that you were likely completely unaware of. Front and center in your efforts to regain lost muscle is to boost the hormone oxytocin, whose release from the brain is under the control of gut microbes. Oxytocin is primarily known as the hor-mone of love and empathy, but it is also *the hormone of body composi-tion*.[5-9] It works to restore youthful muscle mass and strength while helping shrink abdominal visceral fat. Reducing abdominal visceral fat also leads to a reduction in ectopic fat, including fat that accumulates in muscle (myosteatosis), further amplifying the benefits of restoring youthful muscle. Oxytocin also reduces desire for snacking, so-called hedonic eating—eating just for pleasure or indulgence. You will find it easier and easier to pass on the dessert tray or that late-night bowl of ice cream because you simply lose the desire, no exercise of willpower required.

Oxytocin is also the hormone of youthfulness, as it smooths skin wrinkles by restoring youthful facial muscles—no "Ozempic face" here—but also increases dermal collagen, increases libido, increases testosterone in males, increases vaginal moisture and sensation in older females, preserves bone density, and encourages deep sleep. And, because oxytocin is also the hormone of social behavior, you will likely experience more intense feelings of love and affection for the people close to you, increased generosity, reduced anxiety in social settings, and—my favorite—increased acceptance of the opinions of others.[10-11]

Many people have heard that hugging your children or petting a dog boosts oxytocin. But those are transient, momentary effects that are too brief to be of much physiologic benefit—you don't pet your dog and obtain smoother skin or firmer thighs, do you? Instead, we should strive for around-the-clock boosts in oxytocin that we can accomplish by restoring a bacterial microbe that has been lost by nearly all modern humans: *Lactobacillus reuteri*, a.k.a. *L. reuteri*, a microbe whose beneficial effects I discussed in my book *Super Gut*. Despite its importance in so many aspects of health, *L. reuteri* is also susceptible to common antibiotics. For instance, the amoxicillin you were prescribed twenty years earlier for an upper respiratory or bladder infection wiped out all the *L. reuteri* in your GI tract and you therefore lost all its benefits on shape and body composition.[12-14] We'll restore this important microbe in high numbers obtained through fermentation, specifically making something that resembles yogurt but is entirely unlike the anemic version available in grocery stores or made at home using conventional methods. This will enable you to obtain hundreds of billions of microbes, numbers that pack a wallop in beneficial effects.

15 MINUTES, 13 POUNDS

I personally adopted these strategies several years ago when I was in my early sixties. I knew what the scientific evidence showed, but I did not know what to expect in my own personal experience. And my experience was an over-the-top success.

I've made use of my local gym for many years but, in truth, I really don't like going. The whole process of changing into workout clothes, checking in, battling for use of the machines, etc. I'll do anything to minimize my reliance on the facilities. Instead, I'll bike or go for a walk or engage in other activities, relying on the gym facilities only for the resistance-training machines. Because I dislike it, I typically venture into the facility once per week for no more than fifteen to twenty minutes. I do a quick circuit or two of resistance exercises that stress larger muscles, such as quadriceps, latissimus, and shoulders, then hightail it out the front door.

I experimented with adding *Lactobacillus reuteri* to the "yogurt" made by using my method of prolonged fermentation yielding hundreds of billions of microbes per ½-cup serving (far greater numbers than you can obtain through commercial probiotics). I tracked my body composition with a body composition scale (more on how to do this in Appendix D). Over a three-week period, to my surprise, my muscle mass increased by 13 pounds. Strength-wise, I watched the amount of weight I could handle increase by 50 percent over my fifteen to twenty minutes of effort. I had been, for example, doing lat-pulldowns, 130 pounds for ten repetitions, that increased to 200 pounds for ten repetitions—a nearly 50 percent increase over three weeks, fifteen to twenty minutes per week, surely a minimal effort. I regained strength that I hadn't experienced in nearly forty years.

I don't believe that everyone will experience the same magnitude of muscle-restoring effect that I did. One phenomenon I've noticed: People who were more muscular in their youth regain more muscle with the boost in oxytocin provoked by restoration of *L. reuteri*. (I lifted a lot of weights in my teenage years and early twenties.) A former weight lifter or wrestler, for instance, will likely regain more muscle than, say, a long-distance runner. Given what we observed in our recent clinical trial, however, I believe that over 90 percent of people regain muscle lost with aging (and weight loss), but the amount regained varies.

LOST NUTRIENTS

I've discussed how the era of advice to reduce fat intake—total fat, saturated fat, and cholesterol—will be remembered as one of the biggest, most damaging blunders ever made in nutritional thinking that played a major role in creating the current epidemics of overweight, obesity, type 2 diabetes, fatty liver, and other conditions. Along with the proliferation of ultraprocessed foods in the form of chips, shakes, soft drinks, breakfast cereals, and other foods with long, unpronounceable lists of ingredients, the combination proved lethal. This issue alone is enough to fill an entire book, so suffice to say that there never was good evidence to support the idea that reducing fat and cholesterol reduces cardiovascular risk.[15] In fact, a diet with reduced fat and cholesterol makes way for an increase in carbohydrates, especially those sourced from grains and sugars that increase insulin resistance and inflammation, grow abdominal visceral fat, and increase weight. Not limiting fat—for instance, including butter, meats with the fat left on, full-fat ground meats, more extra-virgin olive oil, full-fat dairy, and so on—is also satiating, helping eliminate the always-hungry feeling experienced by people who reduce dietary fat.

As if that wasn't enough, I previously mentioned that three nutrients in particular have nearly disappeared from the modern diet, thanks to the misguided notion of reducing fats and cholesterol, nutrients that play an important role in maintaining muscle and reducing abdominal visceral fat: collagen, hyaluronic acid, and carotenoids such as astaxanthin, factors that synergize to amplify the body-reshaping benefits of *L. reuteri*. Let's explore each of these lost nutrients a little more closely.

Collagen

Increasing intake of collagen alone builds lean muscle mass. This is true for young people, older people, males, and females—in other words, it is a universal phenomenon.[16,17] Restoring collagen intake also makes contributions to reducing insulin resistance and inflammation, thereby accelerating your shape- and body composition–modifying efforts, including loss of abdominal visceral fat.[18] You can, of course, obtain plenty of collagen by adding organ meats back to your diet. Unfortunately, most modern people have become so squeamish over the prospect of adding tongue or heart, coupled with the difficulty of obtaining such foods from the grocery store, that we have the convenient option of obtaining collagen from various commercial powders available. Later in the book, I shall discuss the pros and cons of various sources, dosing, and ways to easily incorporate collagen into your day-to-day routine.

Hyaluronic Acid

Likewise, hyaluronic acid has largely disappeared from the modern diet but, when restored, yields important shape and body-composition effects. But it does so indirectly through beneficial effects on the gastrointestinal microbiome. Recall that hyaluronic acid sourced from animal products is a fiber, which makes it unique in that nearly all other fibers metabolized by gut flora are sourced from plants. Women may be familiar with hyaluronic acid, as it is a popular topical product applied as "serums" to smooth and moisturize skin, or injected as filler into skin to reduce wrinkles. But it yields greater effect when taken *orally* (or with synergistic effects when combined with topical application), as it causes a bloom in beneficial gastrointestinal microbiome species that yield the fatty acid butyrate, which reduces insulin resistance and inflammation, reduces blood glucose, and improves sleep, all adding up to providing beneficial effects in preserving muscle, reducing abdominal visceral fat and thereby fat infiltration of muscle.[19] When consumed orally, hyaluronic acid increases dermal moisture significantly, promotes greater production of collagen in the dermal layer of skin, and causes a modest acidification of the skin that discourages blemishes and rashes.

Carotenoids

I've discussed how carotenoids are yet another casualty of the modern diet. While some carotenoids are sources of vitamin A, such as beta-carotene, another important role of this class of nutrients is to reduce oxidative injury to organs, a process underlying, along with insulin resistance and inflammation, many modern health conditions. The modern shift to ultraprocessed, nutrient-poor foods has resulted in reduced intake of carotenoids of all varieties.[20] Carotenoid intake for most modern people is, unfortunately, dismal. Our return to whole foods that include vegetables and fruits therefore ups your intake of numerous carotenoids.

Six ounces of wild salmon provides 4 mg of astaxanthin. Unfortunately, it is not a good idea to eat salmon every day, as mercury contamination has become an increasingly problematic issue with seafood consumption, due to human activities such as coal burning and mining.

So we turn to supplemental forms of astaxanthin, the carotenoid with the greatest antioxidative potency.[21]

This particular carotenoid poses interesting properties for those of us working to restore youthful body composition. By itself, for instance, astaxanthin supplementation reduces waist circumference by several centimeters, even without changes in diet or exercise, also thereby reducing a major factor in myosteatosis.[22] Astaxanthin also provokes significant anti-inflammatory effects, lowering blood levels of inflammation-mediating compounds and reducing insulin resistance, adding further to its ability to reduce abdominal visceral fat and thereby support a return of youthful muscle. These same inflammatory cytokines, such as NF-κB and TNF-β, are also the suspected mediators of "inflammaging," the increased inflammation that accompanies aging. Astaxanthin is a potent suppressor of the markers for inflammaging, adding to our potential to unwind, or at least slow, many of the phenomena of aging, including age-related muscle loss. Like hyaluronic acid, astaxanthin also helps "mold" the GI microbiome, cultivating blooms in species (such as *Akkermansia*) that further amplify benefits of reducing abdominal fat, reducing waist circumference, maintaining or increasing muscle, and reducing myosteatosis.

The restoration of these three factors largely lost from the modern human dietary experience, especially when combined with restoration of *L. reuteri* to the GI microbiome, provides a powerful and synergistic effect on restoring youthful shape and contours. We'll dive deeper into how they achieve these effects in Chapter 6.

MIRROR, MIRROR: MEASURING YOUR PROGRESS

With the mix of changes that develop following these concepts, how do you track your progress? As abdominal visceral fat recedes, followed by subcutaneous fat, along with increase in muscle mass, not to mention the huge metabolic benefits that develop, how can you measure your gains and losses?

Of course, you could just look in the mirror to observe the reduction in waist size as a flatter abdomen and/or loss of the "love handles" that dangle at the sides. While the mirror cannot tell you how much fat lost from the abdomen is the visceral fat within the abdominal cavity, and how much is subcutaneous just below the skin, the reduction of waist circumference is nonetheless among the most important beneficial features to develop with these efforts. Rest assured that the strategies you adopt in this approach preferentially target loss of the internal fat first. But, at some point, you should also begin to see abdominal muscle peeking through as subcutaneous fat also recedes. You should also begin to see firmness in your shoulders, upper arms, buttocks, thighs, and calves as youthful muscle begins to make a comeback. You'll additionally notice that you are more agile and better able to navigate the world confidently, to climb flights of stairs with greater ease, to handle physically demanding tasks more easily.

While an imperfect method, it can help to measure your waist circumference using an inexpensive cloth tape measure. If you are like most people engaging in these strategies, you are likely to see several inches lost from waist circumference over the initial ninety days, more over a longer time period. Some people lose 6 or more inches over the first ninety days. The key is to make your measurements at roughly the same time of day, at the same level of the abdomen, and to regulate breathing such that you capture your measurement at the end of an exhalation, since you want any changes to be due to reductions in abdominal fat, not in imprecision in measurement. (See Appendix D for the details of reproducibly measuring waist circumference.)

Measuring muscle is not as readily accomplished as measuring abdominal fat. Beyond relying on the mirror, you have another option: Measure gains in muscle using a body composition (bioimpedance) scale. By passing a minor, imperceptible electrical current through your body, this scale measures the varying resistances of fat versus muscle to calculate the quantity of each tissue type. Medical-grade devices that can be found in some doctors' offices or gyms typically pass a current from one hand and one foot through the torso and abdomen, then capture it in the opposite hand and foot. Professional devices also use multiple current frequencies to improve accuracy. Home devices that are more affordable usually pass a current into one foot, then capture it as it exits through the other foot, using a single frequency of electrical current. Home devices are therefore not as accurate, but accuracy for our purposes is not as important as trackability; that is, having a value that we can track as muscle mass increases and fat decreases. These home devices are perfectly adequate for this purpose and can be obtained for less than $100. Some, but not all, bioimpedance devices also add a calculation to estimate the amount of abdominal visceral fat. While not as accurate as, say, CT, MRI, or dual X-ray absorptiometry (DEXA), other methods to gauge body composition, visceral fat values provided by bioimpedance are still useful to track your progress in shrinking abdominal visceral fat. (See Appendix D for a list of recommended devices.)

It can also help to take a photograph at the start of the three-week program, then at the end, and then again at the ninety-day mark. It may be uncomfortable to take that "before" photo, but because the shifts in your shape and body composition unfold gradually, day by day, you are likely to be pleasantly surprised at the often dramatic improvements made over time. And, of course, should you share your before and after photos, you will inevitably inspire others to learn how to favorably alter shape and body composition.

A note about blood work. I advise against having lab work during these efforts, as the processes you are going through introduce confusing changes into your lab values. For instance, as you lose abdominal fat, both visceral and subcutaneous, you are mobilizing triglycerides (i.e., fats) into your bloodstream. If you were to have a standard cholesterol panel drawn, you will see an increase in triglycerides along with a drop in HDL cholesterol (the "good"), since HDL is degraded in the presence of increased triglycerides. You are also likely to see higher blood sugars and even erratic blood pressure readings, as the release of triglycerides can disrupt these measures (causing many physicians, most of whom are unfamiliar with weight-loss phenomena, to make statements like "See, I told you that lifestyle was going to kill you!" or "Now you're going to need a high dose of Lipitor."). But these effects are transient and will eventually improve; there is no need to "treat" these phenomena. If you wait at least several weeks or, preferably, a few months after you have achieved your shape and body composition goals, you are likely to see triglyceride levels of ≤60 mg/dl, HDL cholesterol exceeding 60 mg/dl, fasting blood glucose of 60 to 90 mg/dl. If you were to have the more detailed advanced lipoprotein testing that reveals the real causes of heart disease risk, you are also likely to see that small LDL particles, the actual cause of heart disease, not the outdated and unreliable LDL cholesterol, reach zero—eliminated—or drop to another low value. Not only will you look and feel better, but you will also achieve a level of superior metabolic health.

And you're likely going to endure questions from friends and coworkers who ask, "You must be working out an awful lot, aren't you?" Or "What's different about you—Botox, liposuction?" You're also likely to be first to be chosen for the pickleball team, as you're the one who jumps higher, runs faster, and dives for the ball better than the others, or you're the frequent winner in the doubles tennis game because you play like someone twenty years younger.

LOST AND FOUND

You may have noticed that there are common threads winding throughout all the strategies I am presenting here. There are no pharmaceuticals, no procedures, no nutritional supplements to "treat" some condition. Instead, we are restoring factors that should have been part of human life all along but have been lost or are lacking.

L. reuteri should have been given to you by your mother as you passed through the birth canal at delivery or through breastfeeding. But your mom, like the rest of us, likely lost this microbe because she, too, was exposed to multiple courses of antibiotics that eradicated this microbe. Or you, yourself, were prescribed course after course of antibiotics during your life. As a result of this and other microbiome disruptive factors, nearly all of us have lost this crucial microbe.

The era of "cut your saturated fat and cholesterol" caused unnatural changes in dietary habits. It caused nearly everyone to abandon consumption of organ meats rich in collagen and hyaluronic acid. We therefore restore these long-forgotten nutrients to our shape- and body composition–altering efforts. We then compensate for the reduced carotenoid intake of ultraprocessed modern industrial foods with astaxanthin, the most potent carotenoid of all. Increasing intake of other carotenoids, such as beta-carotene and lutein, is readily accomplished simply by making a return to consumption of real whole foods, such as spinach, lettuces (e.g., red and green leaf), kale, and egg yolks. (You will see these carotenoids figuring prominently in some of the recipes I provide; see pages 201–233.) We therefore amplify the body-shape benefits by adding astaxanthin to the carotenoid mix.

Throw away your calorie-counting tables and apps. Toss all those low-fat cookbooks in the trash. Stock your refrigerator and pantry shelves with fatty meats, poultry and fish with the skin left on, butter and other full-fat dairy; load up on extra-virgin olive oil; then purge the grain and sugar products. Whole grain or white, it makes no difference, as they all exert the same undesirable physiologic effects that distort shape and body composition.

I will be discussing the results of a human clinical trial my team performed in which my recommended combination—*L. reuteri*, collagen peptides, hyaluronic acid, and astaxanthin—were administered to volunteers who were advised to not make any changes in diet or exercise, yet lost an unprecedented quantity of abdominal fat, shrinking their waist circumferences by several inches.

There will be no need to call your health-care insurer to get the go-ahead, no five-figure bills to pay for pharmaceuticals or medical procedures, no emotional breakdowns when you cannot go any further in a demanding exercise program. You can freely go about your business, making a handful of changes in food choices, restoring nutrients lost due to misguided advice to cut fat and cholesterol, and adding a few foods that yield gastrointestinal microbial benefits, and then you can watch your waistline, buttocks, and thighs shrink; see your shoulders stronger and more prominent in a low-cut outfit; your facial features become more firm and pronounced; and walk faster and more proudly compared to your peers.

5

MICROBIOME:
COMMAND CENTER OF MUSCLE
AND BODY COMPOSITION

IN THE PREVIOUS CHAPTER, WE DISCUSSED THE CRUCIAL ROLE of the gut-muscle axis. Let's now consider in greater detail how modern life has damaged the ecosystem that you house within your GI tract—the gastrointestinal microbiome, the trillions of creatures that dwell in the 30 feet of your mouth, esophagus, stomach, duodenum, jejunum, ileum, and colon. These are living creatures that perform myriad beneficial functions for their human host, including playing a role in the gut-muscle axis, a communication system in which microbes communicate with muscle as well as fat. Yes: Microbes play a critical role in the quantity and location of muscle and fat, and you are reliant on them to determine weight, shape, and body composition.

I am continually shocked at the number of people who live their lives struggling with GI complaints, sometimes crippling: bowel urgency, diarrhea, constipation, bloating, often dismissed by their gastroenterologists as neurotic or overreacting symptoms because no ulcer or cancer was seen on their endoscopy. Or they have intolerances to long lists of foods that, when consumed, trigger joint pain, skin rashes, emotional swings, asthma, bloating, or other effects, often leaving them able to consume only a short list of "safe" foods. It all reflects disruption of the microbes inhabiting the modern GI tract, as well as the locations where they have migrated, taking up residence where they do not belong and thereby wreaking a wide range of health havoc. Part of the dietary effort to restore control over shape and body composition must therefore factor in the microbiome's contribution.

A long list of factors unique to modern life—overexposure to antibiotics, food additives, herbicide and pesticide residues in food, and many others—have devastated the human GI microbiome. Literally hundreds of species have been lost, many of which performed crucial functions for the human host. Among the effects lost with these microbes are control over appetite, maintenance of muscle mass, suppression of cortisol (a stress hormone that triggers stress, appetite, and abdominal weight gain), increased depression and anxiety, regulation of insulin responses that determine the location of body fat, and disruption of sleep.

Lost microbes also result in failure to suppress the proliferation of undesirable fecal—yes, fecal—microbes in the GI tract that drive expansion of abdominal fat stores (an important phenomenon that I shall discuss in greater detail later in the book, as it is a major player in determining body composition). All of this adds up to distortions of body shape and composition that, no matter how healthy or meticulous your diet or exercise routine, will cause your body to resist such positive efforts. The solution is therefore not a drug to block some metabolic pathway or a procedure to shrink stomach volume. It's not a sleeping pill to force sleep or an antidepressant drug to increase serotonin. It's certainly not limiting calories or fat. The solution is to restore lost microbes that reshape your body contours, reducing bulges where you don't want them, restoring bulges where you do want them.

In gaining an understanding of the role of the GI microbiome, you may have to suffer through some discussions in which we name specific microbes with tongue-twisting names that play outsize roles in your body, whether you know it or not. Your first thought to aid in the restoration of these microbes may be to take an over-the-counter probiotic, of which there are many. These, however, are not the solution, as such off-the-shelf probiotics are just haphazard collections of microbes that are among the least effective strategies you can adopt to regain control over an errant GI microbiome. Instead, we'll discuss how fermenting foods at room temperature to obtain such microbial species as *Leuconostoc mesenteroides* or *Lactobacillus plantarum* that live on the surface of vegetables and can proliferate as kefir or sauerkraut. We'll discuss how we can ferment human-sourced microbial species as *Lactobacillus reuteri* and *Lactobacillus gasseri* as a food that looks and smells like yogurt (but is not yogurt), microbial species that you should have had occupying your GI tract from the start, obtained from your mom at birth or during infancy, but were eradicated by your exposure to antibiotics and other factors. We'll restore these important bacterial species at high counts, higher than obtainable through a commercial probiotic. Doing so is not just about gastrointestinal health; it is also helpful in restoring or regulating hormones such as insulin, oxytocin, and cortisol that we learned about in the previous chapter. The factors released by the trillions of microbes living and dying in your GI tract determine whether you expand or contract abdominal fat, help determine whether you have fat in your joints or liver, and help determine how much muscle you can flex.

AGING AND THE SHIFTING TIDES OF BODY COMPOSITION

All living creatures age. Along with salamanders, worms, otters, bonobo apes—we all share in this peculiar but fascinating process called aging.

We all recognize the signs of aging in our own species. Beyond an aversion to hip-hop music, we notice thinning skin with wrinkles and age spots, difficulty navigating stairs, reduced flexibility and agility, reduced vigor and strength. But reduced muscle? Age-related loss of muscle is something most of us don't think about much, accepting such changes as just part of the natural and inevitable process of aging. Loss of muscle is one of the most powerful and defining features of aging, and it is largely under the control of not how frequently you visit the gym, not how many Zumba or CrossFit classes you attend, and not whether you indulge in daily protein shakes but microbes living in your GI tract.

I believe that, by now, you can appreciate why we have the world's worst epidemic of overweight, obesity, and unwanted bulges in the history of our species on this planet. Misguided dietary guidelines, an exploitative food industry, lack of nutrients that influence insulin resistance, the loss of body-shaping factors in diet, disruption of the microbiome, and age-related loss of muscle—together are just too much for our bodies to overcome. Doing more of the same is clearly not the answer. We must do something different. And it most definitely should not include injectable drugs or surgical incisions.

This includes taking a long and hard look at the microbes we harbor in our GI tracts, major players in body composition, including preservation or increase in muscle mass. Who would have predicted that microbes, smaller than the head of a pin, too small to see with the naked eye, were the command center for so much of human health and physiology? Could you have imagined that the shape and contours of your body were largely under the control of microscopic creatures? You may have believed that the only other life humans could harbor within themselves were children they became pregnant with. But no, we have trillions of microbes living in our GI tract and other body parts that perform numerous and varied functions. Their importance, however, has only come to be appreciated in the relatively recent past. It's also become clear that, given modern lifestyles, we have negatively affected this microbial world with profound consequences for health and body composition.

I stumbled onto some of these insights by accident when my team and I performed a human clinical trial in an attempt to understand the effects of restoring a microbe lost by most humans, *Lactobacillus reuteri* (*L. reuteri*) that I introduced earlier. The *L. reuteri* story is an entire book in itself, as it is one of the most fascinating and multifaceted microbes that ever found a haven in the human GI tract.

SMOOTHER SKIN . . . BETTER BODY?

I initially focused on *L. reuteri* because of experimental evidence suggesting that it improved various aspects of health and youth, such as enhanced immune response, accelerated healing, prevented weight gain, and increased muscle, and reduced many of the undesirable effects of stress. After I began talking about these effects, and thousands of people began making "yogurt" with this microbe, virtually all the observations made in experimental animals were mirrored in the human experience. (Recall that this is *not* yogurt in the conventional sense, but it looks and smells like yogurt. We ferment it to increase the number of microbes a thousandfold.) Despite these wonderful effects, many of the women in my audience were most interested in the benefits it had on their skin. My team therefore performed a small clinical study, females only, to quantify the skin effects. I combined *L. reuteri* with collagen peptides, hyaluronic acid, and the carotenoid astaxanthin, providing in capsule form those factors that had previously been shown to reduce skin wrinkle depth when consumed individually.

We used such methods as high-resolution skin ultrasound that revealed increased dermal thickness (15%) over ninety days, a result dramatically exceeding the effects, for example, of collagen alone, which typically achieves a 6–7 percent increase in dermal thickness over the same time period. The study also revealed a reduction in skin wrinkles and an increase in skin moisture. Although it was a study of skin effects, we also measured waist circumference. At the start of the study, we asked the twenty-five participants to not make any changes in diet or exercise, only to take the capsules provided for the study. To my surprise, participants lost an average of 7.2 centimeters (nearly 3 inches) off their waist circumference over the ninety days of the study, and as much as 21.6 centimeters (8½ inches) for some of the participants. Even more unexpectedly, despite losing as much as 8½ inches off their waists, there was little reduction in body weight (about ⅓ pound). How could participants lose a profound quantity of abdominal fat, yet not lose weight? Consistent with the animal evidence and with the experiences of the thousands of people in my audience, they likely gained muscle. In short, participants enjoyed a profound shift in body composition.

I detailed my personal experience with this microbe in the previous chapter. In addition to my restored muscle, my chronic insomnia finally passed, and I began to enjoy deep, uninterrupted sleep. I felt less irritated, more compassionate and generous, and the intensity of affection for those close to me was intensified (effects that result from the boost in the brain's release of the hormone oxytocin, which I shall discuss).

L. reuteri has been lost by nearly all modern humans despite being ubiquitous in the GI tracts of hunter-gatherer humans living in the few remaining jungles and savannahs of the planet, as well as all nonhuman mammals studied, all unexposed to antibiotics and other modern factors.[1-3] Its ubiquity suggests that it plays important roles in mammalian health and that its loss poses a major threat, including loss of factors important to shape and body composition.

Through the arguments in *SUPER Body*, I cannot claim that the strategies articulated here will have you rock climbing or mountain biking at age ninety, but I do believe that, given what we now know about this microbe and its effects, we can significantly postpone many of the phenomena of aging by restoring youthful characteristics, including a return of healthy musculature and all its physiological benefits. Restoration of the lost microbe, *L. reuteri*, plays a pivotal role, especially when combined with body-shaping benefits provided by restoring lost nutrients discussed in the last chapter: collagen, hyaluronic acid, and astaxanthin.

How can the restoration of just one microbial species exert such enormous effects on humans? Let's consider that next.

Lois, 61

"IN ADDITION TO THE CALM AND PEACEFULNESS THAT I FELT after about three months of a daily serving of *L. reuteri* Yogurt, I noticed that I felt stronger. I began to 'feel' my muscles in my legs and in my arms, just like when I was younger.

As a result, I started lifting light weights at home. Noticing the loss of belly fat, I became active again. Now, in addition to lifting weights at home, I've started taking fitness classes at the local gym. My increased strength and mobility have changed my mindset about aging. I've not felt, physically and emotionally, this good in years!"

OXYTOCIN: THE HORMONE OF SHAPE AND BODY COMPOSITION

Recall that restoration of *L. reuteri* to the human GI microbiome provokes release of the hormone oxytocin from the brain. This finally addressed a major dilemma that, until now, had no solution: how to boost oxytocin levels throughout the body, around the clock. Previously, the most common way to administer oxytocin was through a nasal inhaler: inserting a device into each nostril, three squirts per nostril every six hours. It's an annoying regimen and one that does not yield full body-wide effects. This has been done, for instance, in autistic children and shown to increase persistence of eye gaze and improve sociability. It's also been administered in couples' therapy to enhance the likelihood of each partner feeling empathy for their partner's point of view. This regimen has been tested in college students given the task of sharing money, with increased generosity after oxytocin inhalation. But these are momentary effects, and no one wants to stick a nozzle up their nose every few hours. The idea that we can restore a microbe to the human GI tract that then triggers your brain to release oxytocin— well, that's revolutionary.

It's an exciting and novel concept: The brain hormone oxytocin, its release triggered by GI microbes, can determine the contours of your body and the location of fat and muscle. Trillions of tiny creatures, anonymous and largely unappreciated, play a major role in determining your waist size, whether you have fat in your buttocks or thighs, whether you maintain youthful musculature, how easily you can climb a flight of stairs or swing a golf club, the quality of your social interactions, and the intensity of affection you feel for other human beings.

Researchers have been exploring the question of hormonal influences over body shape issues for well over a century. Why do some people accumulate fat in the abdomen, yet others accumulate it in the hips and thighs? Why can some people succumb to health issues that can be blamed on excessive loss of muscle (sarcopenia), while others do not?

We know, for instance, that an excess of the adrenal hormone cortisol, as occurs with prolonged stress or taking a related prescription form of the hormone, such as prednisone, can cause abdominal visceral fat to explode in quantity while causing muscle atrophy. Yes, emotional stress can be a major factor in the size of your waist, accelerate age-related loss of muscle, and amplify the negative effects of excess weight, adding insult to injury. We also know that lack of testosterone in an aging male will decrease muscle mass and strength and increase abdominal fat. There's also the increasingly common situation in which excess insulin provoked by cortisol and an unhealthy diet drives accumulation of abdominal visceral fat while also causing fat to be deposited in ectopic locations such as muscle, the heart, pancreas, knees, and hips.

The hormone oxytocin that originates from the brain was believed by most to be nothing more than the hormone of love and empathy, transiently triggered by hugging your child or petting a dog. Or viewed as a hormone administered intravenously at term pregnancy to provoke uterine contraction and delivery of a newborn baby. The notion that it might exert major influence on the shape of your body or its composition is completely foreign to most people, including most doctors. But the emerging evidence of the past decade does indeed suggest that oxytocin is a neglected yet incredibly powerful factor that determines the location of fat and muscle, body shape, as well as skin appearance, joint health, posture, vigor, and thereby youthfulness. Beyond direct effects of oxytocin itself, restoring *L. reuteri*, and thereby oxytocin, also exerts major positive effects on cortisol, testosterone, insulin, and other body shape–determining hormones. And, incredibly, the quantity of oxytocin released by the brain is largely under the control—not of diet, not exercise, not pharmaceuticals, not how often you pet your dog—of *microbes* dwelling in the gastrointestinal tract. Yes: Microbes that live and die in the 30 feet of your GI tract, mouth to anus, are the principal determinants of your shape and body composition. Microbes that you empty into the toilet every day as a pound or two of fecal material are the stars in the movie that is your life, shape, and body composition.

THE NUCLEAR WINTER OF OUR MICROBIOME

I've discussed how numerous dietary blunders have been made in the era of "cut your fat, cut your cholesterol," such as increased reliance on ultraprocessed foods that raise blood sugar and add to risk for type 2 diabetes and weight gain, the widespread addition of such unhealthy additives as preservatives and emulsifying agents, and abandonment of organ meats and thereby intake of collagen and hyaluronic acid. These perversions of the natural human dietary script alone are enough to significantly distort shape and body composition, cause weight gain, and expand abdominal visceral and ectopic fat, amplifying loss of muscle over that from aging alone while also accelerating many of the phenomena of aging, such as increased skin wrinkles, deterioration of joints, and unhealthy effects on the brain that increase potential for cognitive decline and dementia.

The situation was hugely worsened by the unrestrained intake of antibiotics that decimate the GI microbiome. Over 1,300 prescriptions for antibiotics are dispensed every year, for instance, for every one thousand children. One in three adults receives an antibiotic prescription every year, a practice that kills off trillions of microbes, many beneficial, in our GI tracts with each and every exposure.[4] In the century since the first antibiotic, penicillin, was discovered, antibiotics have become as commonplace as blue jeans or smartphones, prescriptions dispensed by doctors at the slightest provocation: a cough, fever, or body ache, whether or not the cause is bacterial. And many antibiotics are "broad spectrum"; that is, they kill a wide range of microbes. As a result, GI microbiomes of twenty-first-century humans are unlike the

GI microbiomes of pre-antibiotic generations. Compare the modern GI microbiome of someone in, say, New York or Los Angeles with that of humans unexposed to antibiotics living in the Brazilian rainforest or jungles of New Guinea. Hunter-gatherer humans who hunt and forage for food without exposure to antibiotics or other modern factors have in their GI tracts hundreds of microbial species that we have lost.[5,6] Just as a nuclear bomb dropped on a population indiscriminately kills children, women, men, the sick, the well, teachers, shopkeepers, maintenance men, college professors, lawyers, accountants, and so on, so do antibiotics kill microbes without concern for whether they were necessary, leaving a virtual nuclear winter of destruction. Among the most critical casualties: *L. reuteri*.

Examine the GI microbiomes of mammals living in the wild (none of which is overweight or obese): They all have *L. reuteri*. Study the GI microbiome of slender, muscled free-living humans dwelling in the highland jungles of New Guinea or the Amazonian rainforest, hunting or gathering their next meal: They, too, all have *L. reuteri*. Despite its ubiquity in all mammals and indigenous human populations unexposed to antibiotics and other antimicrobial factors, nearly all modern people have lost this microbe. You can't help avoiding the conclusion that this microbe is therefore essential for the health and shape of mammals, including *Homo sapiens*—and we have lost it.

L. reuteri, as well as many other potentially beneficial species of the human microbiome, is susceptible to common antibiotics. Although antibiotics are sometimes necessary, we cannot escape the fact that they are indiscriminate: They kill the bad, such as *Pneumococcus*, which causes a debilitating and sometimes deadly form of pneumonia, or the *E. coli* that is a frequent cause of urinary infections. But antibiotics also kill the good. A single course of an antibiotic means that, in the microbial warfare waged by taking an antibiotic, beneficial GI microbes are the casualties of friendly fire. In other words, the antibiotic you were prescribed years ago for a bladder or sinus infection wiped out all the *L. reuteri* in your gut.

German microbiologist Dr. Gerhard Reuter discovered this microbe in 1962, isolated from the breast milk of a breastfeeding mother. In the ensuing forty years of his academic career, Dr. Reuter found it increasingly difficult to recover this microbe from human body secretions. More recent assessments of the human microbiome have corroborated Dr. Reuter's struggle: *L. reuteri* has almost completely disappeared from the modern human microbiome, no longer recoverable in breast milk, the GI tract, or bowel movements. The antibiotics that you may have taken long ago wiped out the populations of this microbe in your body, and with its loss, all the spectacular benefits this one microbial species provided to humans.

Drawing from a combination of animal and human evidence, we know that restoration of this lost microbe is associated with numerous health benefits, many of them driven by provoking release of the hormone oxytocin. Benefits of oxytocin relevant to body shape and composition include:

- Restoration of youthful muscle and strength—Recall that we lose about 30 percent of youthful muscle as we age, a major determining factor in posture, gait, and contours of our body, as well as a factor influencing metabolic health and ability to control weight. This effect appears to depend on the degree of musculature you enjoyed in your younger years: The more muscled you were, the more muscle returns under influence of oxytocin. But even nonathletes enjoy restoration of former musculature.[7,8] In our own human clinical trial experience, fat can be lost while preserving or increasing muscle, a phenomenon that can be expected to prevent regain of fat weight in the long term.
- Reduction of cortisol—Many people suffer from chronic stress. Stress can originate with work, family, money, and other modern struggles that, for many, is a 24/7 phenomenon. Stress provokes release of greater quantities of the stress hormone cortisol from the adrenal glands that, in turn, increases abdominal and ectopic fat while accelerating muscle atrophy. The oxytocin boost provoked by *L. reuteri* reduces high levels of cortisol back to a more desirable range, thereby giving you further control over body composition.[7] Later in this chapter, I shall discuss another

microbe, *L. gasseri*, also reduced or lost from the human GI tract, which can add to this cortisol-reducing effect and thereby further protect you from inappropriate surges in cortisol.

- Reduced insulin resistance—Recall that poor responsiveness of the body's organs to insulin is a major driver of weight gain, especially in abdominal visceral fat, as well as a major risk factor for coronary heart disease, cognitive decline and dementia, prediabetes and type 2 diabetes, and many forms of cancer. *L. reuteri* reduces insulin resistance, thereby facilitating weight loss from the abdomen and reducing ectopic fat, including myosteatosis, while also reducing risk for so many common modern health conditions.[9]
- Increased testosterone in males—restoring levels in older males back to youthful levels. This also helps restore muscle mass, reduce abdominal fat, and restore a sense of confidence and control.[10]
- Reduction of the snacking impulse—Snacking, or so-called hedonic eating, eating just for pleasure and not to meet physiological need, is the downfall for many people, unable to resist the chips, cookies, ice cream, and other "goodies." The oxytocin boost you obtain by restoring *L. reuteri* reduces this impulse.[11]

The oxytocin boost from *L. reuteri* has other beneficial effects, such as increasing dermal collagen and thereby smoothing skin wrinkles, as we observed in our human clinical trial in which dermal thickness was increased. It also increases libido, as well as the intensity of love and empathy for those close to you, and improves the immune system response.[12] These effects may not improve body shape, but they improve your overall health and well-being. In short, oxytocin makes you a better human being, certainly one better able to navigate all the ups and downs of life, as well as manage the various bulges of body shape.

L reuteri, in addition to provoking oxytocin, has another unique capacity shared by few other microbial species with additional benefits for health and body shape. Not only does *L. reuteri* provoke oxytocin release from the brain, but it also takes up residence in the small intestine (i.e., not just the colon or large intestine), where it produces bacteriocins, natural peptide antibiotics effective against unhealthy, mostly fecal, species in the small intestine where they don't belong.[13] This peculiar situation is called small intestinal bacterial overgrowth (SIBO), in which the 24 feet of stomach, duodenum, jejunum, and ileum are invaded by fecal microbes meant only to live in the colon. Fecal microbes in the small intestine live and die over just a few hours, meaning trillions of microbes turn over rapidly, shedding their components. One of their components is called lipopolysaccharide endotoxin, or just endotoxin, because it is extremely toxic, even in minor quantities. When all this occurs in the small intestine—a segment of the GI tract that is, by design, permeable to allow absorption of nutrients— endotoxin is able to enter the bloodstream, a process called endotoxemia. Endotoxemia due to overgrowth of fecal microbes in the small intestine is a major driver of insulin resistance that promotes expansion of abdominal fat, loss of muscle, and ectopic fat deposition in muscle.

How common is SIBO and its accompanying endotoxemia? Frighteningly common; by my estimation, it is one of the largest epidemics ever in the history of our species. But it is something you can take steps to manage and correct and thereby enjoy reduction or elimination of numerous common health struggles. More on that later.

In short, fecal microbes living where they don't belong underlie the accumulation of abdominal fat and all its associated health problems. Restoration of *L. reuteri* provides major advantages in counteracting this effect by colonizing the full length of the small intestine, as well as the colon, and producing natural antibiotics effective against fecal microbes. The twofold effect of *L. reuteri*—provocation of increased oxytocin release and reduced endotoxemia—make it a crucial factor in regaining control over body shape and composition.

LACTOBACILLUS REUTERI: BODY-MOLDING MICROBE

From the perspective of body composition, by losing *L. reuteri*, you thereby have lost the ability to enjoy a higher level of oxytocin that maintained youthful muscle. You also lost this microbe's ability to discourage overproliferation of fecal microbes in the small intestine that, as a result, caused endotoxemia and thereby insulin resistance that expanded abdominal fat. You also lost the cortisol-reducing, testosterone-boosting, and insulin resistance–reducing effects of oxytocin. Add all these factors together and you have lost the "brake" on weight gain and control over how fat and muscle are distributed.

Restoring *L. reuteri* is therefore the cornerstone of an effort to regain control over shape and body composition. Not only can youthful muscle return, but fecal microbes are pushed back down to the colon where they belong, and the obesity-driving effects of insulin resistance, high cortisol levels, and inflammation are reduced, allowing abdominal visceral and ectopic fat to be released. Appetite is reduced by the unique effect of oxytocin to reduce the desire to snack, sleep is deeper and longer, the immune response is improved, libido increases, testosterone in males increases, and skin is moister and smoother—combined effects that cause many people to receive compliments on how much younger they look and deny that they underwent plastic surgery or had Botox or filler injections.

Think of it: A self-reproducing tiny bacterium that has likely been an inhabitant of the human body for millions of years is now lost, and with it, all its physiological advantages. Given its wonderful effects on human life, this single microbe also probably played an important role in making human life what it is—or was.

Loss of this microbe has likely played a significant role in creating the body distortions that, over the past fifty years, have become all too familiar. Could it have also played a role in such phenomena as an increase in gastrointestinal diseases, emotional struggles (e.g., depression and suicide), and the rise in narcissistic behavior? Sum up the evidence in its entirety, and I believe we could argue that the growing numbers of angry, unsatisfied, socially disconnected, weaker, and fatter humans of the twenty-first century are due, in large part, to the betrayal that we have inflicted on this long-standing accompaniment and friend of human life, *L. reuteri*.

I don't believe that it is a stretch to say that loss of this crucial microbe is tantamount to loss of a hand or eye: You will be impaired for life, struggling to compensate for this disability. And what if the loss of this microbe that has such heavy influence over the body's distribution of muscle and fat also reduces control over impulses such as anger and hate—how many of your health, emotional, and social struggles over your lifetime can be blamed on the loss of this incredible and multipotent microbe?

Mai, 50

"I HAVE SO MUCH MORE ENERGY AND I AM MUCH STRONGER and have way more stamina. I wake up without an alarm clock now. More optimism and more hopeful. More patient and tolerant.

"Hair no longer falls out and is thicker. My eyes are brighter and whiter. No more bleeding gums.

"I sleep better and I have more vivid dreams. Vision has improved.

"Skin complexion is better, the dryness of the legs and elbows has disappeared. The horizontal lines on the nails have disappeared, the nails are now smooth. Before, there were patches of pigment spots on the stomach, under the breast and on the back. They have disappeared. I have a nice, calm, satisfied feeling in my stomach.

"No more joint stiffness in the morning, no more achy knees."

———

That's just one microbe. Should you encounter an indigenous hunter-gatherer human, recognize that, not only is this person unacquainted with your technological insights, they are also microbially distinct, more fully muscled with flat abdomens, and for the most part, maintain good health for the full course of their lifetimes, an experience unfamiliar to any inhabitant of your local assisted living center or nursing home.

WHAT'S A NICE MICROBE LIKE YOU DOING IN A PLACE LIKE THIS?

The human colon, or large intestine, is the most distal 4- to 5-foot-long portion of the GI tract responsible for reabsorbing water and then holding the remains of prior meals to release when the time is appropriate, and not when you are chasing an animal to kill for dinner or courting a potential mate. The colon is also the place where the majority of GI microbes are meant to reside. The likes of *E. coli*, *Salmonella*, and *Campylobacter* are well suited to inhabiting the human colon, as is the colon to housing such residents. Just as squirrels are perfectly comfortable living in trees and salmon are happy to swim upstream, so most microbes that constitute human fecal material are happy in the colon, with its high pH and other factors, and the colon manages just fine housing trillions of microbial inhabitants for the several hours, sometimes days, before they make their happy exit.

But a peculiar situation has emerged in modern humans. Overexposure to antibiotics, preservatives and emulsifying food additives, synthetic sweeteners such as aspartame and sucralose, anti-inflammatory drugs, chlorinated drinking water, and numerous other factors have reduced or killed off microbes in the GI tract that ordinarily suppressed colonic fecal microbes.[14] Unsuppressed, colonic microbes are—remarkably—able to ascend up the 24 feet of small intestine, the situation I mentioned earlier—small intestinal bacterial overgrowth (SIBO).[15] The small intestine is not equipped to deal with trillions of fecal microbes and lacks the defenses that the colon has. The small intestine, for example, has a fragile single-layer barrier of mucus, not the thicker and more protective two-layer mucus barrier of the colon. The small intestine is also, by design, permeable, as this is where the body is meant to absorb amino acids, fatty acids, vitamins, and minerals. When colonic fecal microbes invade the small intestine, you become a sitting duck, allowing breakdown products of fecal microbes to enter the bloodstream. One component, in particular, that of fecal microbes' cell walls called lipopolysaccharide endotoxin, a.k.a. endotoxin, which I mentioned earlier, is released in large quantities and, given the natural permeability of the small intestine, enters the bloodstream, thereby causing endotoxemia. Endotoxemia is a major trigger of insulin resistance, inflammation, cortisol, and other factors that expand abdominal visceral and ectopic fat while impairing muscle.[16]

When fecal microbes invade the small intestine from the colon, health—and body shape—havoc results. Fecal microbes live for only a few hours, not the years of larger creatures. It means that trillions of fecal microbes inhabiting the small intestine, living and dying in rapid succession, release their by-products into the bloodstream. SIBO and the accompanying endotoxemia are unnatural and, given the factors that cause these phenomena, uniquely modern. And they are also occurring with epidemic frequency.

Restoring *L. reuteri*, with its unique capacity to colonize the small intestine and produce bacteriocins that kill invading fecal microbes, is therefore a major first step in reducing these body composition-distorting effects while improving skin and libido, restoring muscle, and providing numerous other health benefits. "Move more, eat less," "push the plate away"—come on, don't make me laugh. Know that, by gaining an understanding of the role of microbes in your shape and body composition, you have achieved a level of understanding light-years ahead of the doctor, dietitian, or dietary guideline.

The unique method I've been using to generate high counts of *L. reuteri* can be found in Appendix B.

THE EPIDEMIC BENEATH OUR NOSES

Modern people are no strangers to epidemics and pandemics: COVID-19, influenza, HIV, type 2 diabetes, etc. Such phenomena fill headlines, prompt lavish parties at pharmaceutical companies for all the new revenue opportunities they provide, and keep doctors and hospitals busy.

But an epidemic of SIBO and endotoxemia—really? Ask most doctors and they typically respond with "Did you consult

Dr. Google again?" Or "There's nothing wrong with you." Or "It's all in your head."

So, why do I make the claim that SIBO and endotoxemia are epidemic, one of the largest and widespread epidemics in the history of our species, bigger than even the epidemics of obesity and type 2 diabetes? Simple: Examine the evidence in which this question was asked:

In condition _____, what proportion of people test positive for SIBO?

(In most studies, breath hydrogen gas testing is used, a method that takes advantage of the fact that microbes produce hydrogen gas, but humans do not. I shall discuss this issue at greater length later in the book, including how to accomplish this in the comfort of your home without a doctor or lab. The proportion testing positive varies with the populations studied and the method used, but this gives you an idea of how common this situation is.)

Let's insert various health conditions into the blank:

Obesity—Of the 108 million obese adults in the United States, about 50 percent test positive, with some studies finding nearly 90 percent.[17,18] That's at least 54 million Americans with SIBO.

Type 2 diabetes—Of the 35 million Americans with type 2 diabetes, 29 percent (10 million) of diabetic Americans have SIBO.[19] Of the more than 90 million Americans with prediabetes, this adds further to the total number (though not yet formally quantified).

Fatty liver—More than 100 million Americans have fatty liver. Add another 35 percent (35 million) of people to the list.[20]

Irritable bowel syndrome (IBS)—Of the 60 to 70 million Americans with IBS, multiple studies demonstrate that 31 percent (19 million) test positive for SIBO, with some estimates as high as 84 percent.[21,22] Add another 20 or so million Americans to our growing list.

Parkinson's disease—Of the nearly one million Americans with this neurodegenerative condition, 52 percent (around 500,000) test positive.[23]

Alzheimer's dementia—Of the 6 million Americans with Alzheimer's dementia, 49 percent (around 3 million) test positive.[24] These numbers don't include the millions of people with earlier forms of cognitive impairment, many of whom also likely have SIBO.

Restless leg syndrome—Of the 30 million Americans with this disruptive sleep disorder, 69 percent (20 million) test positive.[25]

Sleep apnea—Of the 39 million Americans with this condition, 31 percent (12 million) test positive for SIBO.[26]

Tally up the numbers of those testing positive for SIBO, add the numbers of Americans with other neurological conditions, autoimmune diseases, coronary heart disease, inflammatory bowel diseases (ulcerative colitis and Crohn's disease), depression and other mental health conditions, and the many diseases in which testing for SIBO has not yet been performed, and you can appreciate that the numbers of people affected are staggering, easily exceeding 100 million people, or 1 in 3 Americans, and likely more than 150 million. Obviously, there can be overlap among groups, an obese type 2 diabetic, for instance, with fatty liver. But the takeaway message here is that SIBO and its accompanying endotoxemia are exceptionally common, with well over 100 million Americans harboring fecal microbes in their small intestines that allow endotoxemia to add to their health and body composition woes.

We are not talking about a situation that is uncommon. We are talking about a condition that crosses all economic, educational, and racial barriers; affects the young and old, male and female, and residents of every state; and can be present whether you have numerous overt health problems or none. Don't be surprised, however, if your doctor is completely in the dark and has no idea what you are talking about when you raise the question of SIBO. Or they, at best, will hand you a prescription for rifaximin, an antibiotic that is only 55–60 percent effective, costly, and with the expected side effects of antibiotics. But if antibiotics are a big part of the reason that we develop SIBO in the first place, does it make any sense to take yet another antibiotic?

MICROBES LOVE COMPANY

Human beings are social creatures. Most of us thrive in the presence of family, friends, neighbors, coworkers, community. Few of us want to live our lives in isolation. In fact, isolation can be used as a form of torture or punishment in prisons and in war because it defies a basic human instinct.

They may not throw neighborhood parties, they may not be members of your local homeowners' association, but most microbes also do best as members of a community. Our star microbe, *L. reuteri*, is no different. But, given current scientific insights, no one yet knows who are the closest "friends" of this microbe; that is, which microbes, when accompanying *L. reuteri*, help it take up permanent residence. When we restore *L. reuteri* through a probiotic or our yogurt or other fermentation projects, we restore it for no more than about seven days, then it's gone. But why? Likely due to the lack of having restored *L. reuteri*'s "community" of supportive microbes. Perhaps we will, in a few years, come to understand *L. reuteri*'s needs and provide the several microbes it requires to sustain its presence in the human GI tract. Until those insights are uncovered through continued research efforts, are there microbial species that we know could amplify some of the benefits of our lone *L. reuteri*, especially those that provide advantages in our body composition–improving efforts?

Yes, there are two that stand out: *Lactobacillus gasseri* and *Bacillus coagulans*. Let's now consider these two "friends" of *L. reuteri*.

THE GUT-MUSCLE AXIS COMMUNITY

L. reuteri alone is a powerful factor when restored to the human GI tract. Its unique properties of oxytocin provocation, small intestinal colonization, and bacteriocin production make you wonder how we got along without it these last several decades.

You may have heard about the ways the GI microbiome interacts with the various parts of the body: the gut-brain axis, the gut-skin axis, and others. Let's now consider the gut-*muscle* axis, a bidirectional "cross talk" between the GI microbiome and the muscles of the body.[27] Microbes in the GI tract affect how much muscle mass you maintain as well as strength. Muscle use, via exercise or strenuous labor, also exerts effects on the GI microbiome. Most attention has been focused, however, on microbes in the colon that participate in the gut-muscle axis. Instead, we are going to focus on microbes that occupy the small intestine, a location where larger beneficial effects on body composition are exerted.

Compared to the colon, the small intestine is normally a microbial desert. The colon is densely populated, while the 24 feet of small intestine is, under normal conditions, thinly populated. A few microbes from the mouth, for instance, that survived the harsh conditions posed by stomach acid and bile, and a few microbes that ascended from the colon can normally occupy the small intestine. But the small intestine should be like a small farm town in rural America: a feed store, a pharmacy, a few hundred residents, maybe a school, but that's it—a far cry from densely populated urban centers.

When our small rural farm town is invaded by thousands of unwanted visitors, they easily overwhelm resources, especially if there is no sheriff, no police force, no angry vigilantes to defend the town. That is the situation in your duodenum, jejunum, and ileum, the 24 feet of small intestine that is relatively defenseless and invaded by trillions of unwanted fecal visitors from the colon.

L. reuteri therefore comes to the rescue with its unique ability to take up residence in the small intestine and produce bacteriocins that kill invading fecal microbes. But wouldn't you feel better if this

lone microbe had reinforcements, other microbial species that add to
L. reuteri's ability to push back the onslaught of fecal microbes, thereby
reducing endotoxin release and endotoxemia? Providing *L. reuteri*
with microbial reinforcements could mean that you are given even
greater control over health and body contours. Let's now consider the
two microbial species that we know add to the beneficial effects of
L. reuteri.

Lactobacillus gasseri

Add *L. gasseri* to the list of microbes that are now largely reduced
or absent from the human adult GI microbiome, along with other *Lactobacillus* species.[28]

L. gasseri is one of the few beneficial microbial species that, like
L. reuteri, also has the ability to colonize the 24 feet of small intestine.
And, like *L. reuteri*, *L. gasseri* is a powerhouse of bacteriocin production.[29] The unique combination of small intestinal colonization and
bacteriocin production make this microbe an important player in preventing the unhealthy proliferation of fecal microbial species in the
small intestine—SIBO. Restoring the combination of *L. reuteri* and
L. gasseri is therefore an extremely powerful strategy to push back fecal
microbes. (It makes you wonder whether the loss of these two species may be at least part of how and why SIBO has reached epidemic
proportions.) *L. gasseri* has also been demonstrated—on its own—to
shrink waist circumference and reduce abdominal visceral fat, amplifying *L. reuteri*'s beneficial effects.[30] *L. gasseri* also adds to the cortisol-
suppressing properties of *L. reuteri*, blunting the surge in cortisol that
can result from, say, a letter from the IRS or an unpleasant interaction
with your boss, effects that have potential for expanding abdominal
visceral fat and eroding muscle.[31]

Know that, by restoring these two microbial species, you not only
take back control over a wide swath of health phenomena, including
improved GI health, but you are also given enormous control over the
various facets of shape and body composition.

Bacillus coagulans

B. coagulans is different from the other two microbes in that it is consumed as a spore, a hibernating seedlike form, which germinates in the small intestine upon consumption. It is also unique in that it is the only microbe among the three that is found not only in the GI tract of humans and other mammals but also in soil and on the surface of plants, including vegetables. Like the other two species, it also produces bacteriocins effective in eradicating invading fecal microbes in the small intestine.[32] This effect likely explains why many people with irritable bowel syndrome obtain partial or complete relief with supplementation of this microbe.[33]

Relevant to our body composition interests, emerging evidence also suggests that *B. coagulans* is another microbe that participates in the gut-muscle axis, having been shown to restore significant muscle mass while also increasing strength.[34-36] Although the means by which *B. coagulans* achieves this effect is still being explored, at least part of the effect is due to an improvement in the absorption of proteins from the diet, the building blocks of muscle.

Microbes therefore provide considerable advantage in regaining muscle lost with aging, preventing muscle loss with weight loss, and thereby maintaining a favorable BMR and preventing weight regain.

The combination of all three microbes, fermented together using my method of prolonged fermentation (36 hours), is surprisingly effective in eradicating SIBO. Ferment all three together as something that looks and smells like "yogurt"—but is not yogurt—and it has proved to be surprisingly effective in eradicating invading fecal microbes in the small intestine, thereby eradicating SIBO. Let's discuss that idea next.

DO YOU HAVE SIBO?

How do you know whether you are among the one in two or three Americans who have fecal microbes invading the 24 feet of small intestine? One way is to test for hydrogen (H_2) gas on the breath, since microbes produce H_2 but you do not. If you consume a food that microbes convert to H_2 within ninety minutes of consumption, it signifies the presence of fecal microbes in the small intestine, since ninety minutes is too brief a time for the food to reach the colon where H_2 production is normal and expected. In other words, fecal microbes living where they are supposed to live—the colon—normally produce H_2 gas while the small number of microbes living in a healthy small intestine should not. But when fecal microbes come to inhabit the small intestine, they will produce H_2 gas soon after consumption of something they metabolize such as various fibers. For this reason, we use the fiber, inulin, as a powder, ingested in your morning coffee or other food to assess how fast H_2 gas is produced. If, say, you detect H_2 gas on the breath thirty to forty-five minutes after consuming the inulin, then you have fecal microbes infesting your small intestine. Any positive H_2 measurement within ninety minutes after consumption is therefore an indicator of SIBO. Positive measurements after ninety minutes at, say, more than two hours are indeterminate as we cannot distinguish SIBO in the ileum (the most distal part of the small intestine) from normal colonic H_2 production.

In years past, this sort of testing could only be conducted in a laboratory or health clinic: cumbersome, costly, and time-consuming, with few doctors aware of the significance of this testing. Thankfully, we now have a consumer device, the AIRE device, which you can use to measure H_2 gas in the comfort of your home with results obtained within minutes, no co-pay or doctor's order needed. Unlike performing this test in a lab or clinic, purchase the device ($150–$200) once and it can be used over and over again. (See Appendix C for the protocol I use for AIRE testing.) It can be useful to identify SIBO and also in the future to assess whether some symptom signifies recurrence. This can be important because, while the initial symptoms of SIBO may be something like excessive gas or bloating, recurrence months later could be different, such as anxiety or a panic attack. This is because the microbial species responsible can change over time, yielding a different constellation of symptoms.

Although the AIRE device can be helpful in identifying SIBO, you don't necessarily have to purchase the device to know whether you have fecal microbes inhabiting your small intestine. You can also identify SIBO with certainty if any of the following are present:

- Food intolerances—Unpleasant symptoms, such as excessive gas, bloating, abdominal discomfort, rashes, asthma, dark thoughts, anxiety, panic attacks, and so on, after consuming various foods, especially if occurring within the first 90 minutes after consumption, are a solid indicator that you have SIBO causing the intolerance. Intolerances to nightshades (e.g., eggplant, tomatoes), histamine-containing foods (e.g., cheese, wine), fruit, and FODMAPs (fermentable oligosaccharides, disaccharides, monosaccharides and polyols, essentially fibers and sugars), all represent SIBO.[37-39] The solution is therefore not avoidance of these foods; addressing the SIBO causing the intolerance is the answer, freeing you from both the food intolerances as well as numerous other health difficulties.

- Fat malabsorption—Fecal microbes that have invaded the duodenum (just beyond the stomach) block the action of pancreatic digestive enzymes and bile, interfering with digestion of fats. Fats therefore are undigested and pass into the toilet, causing fat droplets to float at the top or fat staining where the water meets the porcelain.[37]

- Irritable bowel syndrome (IBS)—Bowel urgency, diarrhea, and bloating of IBS are highly suggestive of SIBO.[40] (This is why conventional doctors now "treat" IBS with the antibiotic rifaximin.)

- Hypochlorhydria—Low stomach acid that manifests as difficulty or slowed digestion of meats means that you have lost the capacity to produce hydrochloric acid that begins the process of protein digestion. Loss of stomach acid opens the door to infestation from swallowed oral microbes and the ascent of fecal microbes. People who have taken stomach acid–blocking drugs, especially proton pump inhibitors, such as omeprazole, pantoprazole, or esomeprazole, likewise have a high likelihood of SIBO.[41,42]

- History of opioid use—The slowed intestinal action experienced as constipation when taking opioid drugs increases the likelihood that fecal microbes have proliferated and ascended into the small intestine.[42]
- History of nonsteroidal anti-inflammatory drug (NSAID) use—Such drugs as ibuprofen, naproxen, sulindac, and others increase the likelihood of developing SIBO.[43]
- Hypothyroidism—The slowed intestinal activity of hypothyroidism can allow SIBO to develop. Some evidence suggests that people who are prescribed the T4 thyroid hormone (levothyroxine) alone without the T3 thyroid hormone are also at increased risk of developing SIBO.[44,45]

There are other conditions that are so highly associated with SIBO that it is safe to assume it is present and you can therefore take action to eradicate. These conditions include obesity and overweight, type 2 diabetes, fatty liver, fibromyalgia, inflammatory bowel disease, neurodegenerative diseases, autoimmune diseases, restless leg syndrome, sleep apnea, and skin rashes, especially rosacea and psoriasis.[46-51]

Consider this: If the solution to SIBO was something drastic or invasive, say, surgical removal of the small intestine, then we need to be absolutely certain that SIBO is indeed present. But what if the solution for SIBO is something that looks and smells like yogurt that you make in your kitchen that, in addition to wiping out invading fecal microbes in the small intestine, also makes you happier and more generous, smooths skin wrinkles, restores youthful muscle, increases libido, and generates better sleep? Because it is so benign and is accompanied by so many wonderful benefits, you don't need to be absolutely certain that SIBO is present. In fact, you can restore the three microbes of SIBO Yogurt anytime, anywhere.

"SIBO YOGURT"

While you can obtain spectacular shape and body composition benefits by fermenting *L. reuteri* alone, you can also ferment *L. reuteri* with its two "friends," *L. gasseri* and *B. coagulans*, to make something I call SIBO Yogurt, which has been unexpectedly successful in eradicating SIBO in the majority of people who consume it. For example, around 90 percent of people who test positive for hydrogen gas, using the AIRE device, normalize this measure after consuming the SIBO Yogurt for four weeks (longer in severe cases), accompanied by reversal of associated phenomena, such as food intolerances, a break in a weight-loss plateau, or symptoms of bloating and diarrhea, as well as normalization of breath H_2.

Say you took an off-the-shelf probiotic—will SIBO go away? Will the probiotic eradicate the trillions of fecal microbes that have invaded your 24 feet of small intestine? No, it may reduce bloating or diarrhea a bit, but more than likely you will be left with SIBO. But what if we chose species and strains of microbes that (1) colonize the small intestine, since that is where SIBO occurs, and (2) are known to produce bacteriocins effective in killing fecal microbes? I therefore chose the three you are now familiar with: *L. reuteri*, *L. gasseri*, and *B. coagulans*. (Suggested sources can be found in Appendix B.)

Most people normalize breath H_2 by consuming the SIBO Yogurt for four weeks, ½ cup (120 ml) per day (providing around 300 billion microbes per serving). An occasional person who has a severe case of SIBO, such as someone who was prescribed numerous courses of antibiotics over the years, may require several months of consumption to eradicate SIBO. Also, if you test with the AIRE device at the start and would like to assess whether H_2 has been normalized after a course of the SIBO Yogurt, you will have to stop the yogurt for two weeks, then test. This is because *L. reuteri* produces H_2 gas and you won't be able to tell whether you have eradicated SIBO or not. If you don't have an AIRE device, you can track whatever phenomenon that caused you to believe you had SIBO in the first place. If, for example, you developed headaches when consuming eggs, or a panic attack when eating legumes, or witnessed fat malabsorption in the toilet, you will likely experience relief from these effects when SIBO has been reversed. With food intolerances, sample a small serving to see whether the effect is gone, then advance to resuming full serving size if intolerance is not provoked by the test sample.

Be aware that, when you consume the SIBO Yogurt (or any other microbe-eradicating strategy), you can experience the phenomenon of die-off, such as nausea, headaches, fatigue, depression, skin rashes, asthma, nightmares, and other effects that result from the flood of breakdown products into the intestines and bloodstream as fecal microbes die, representing a transient increase in endotoxemia. In other words, it is a sign of success in reducing the burden of fecal microbes. You can reduce the intensity of these unpleasant feelings by reducing the serving size of the SIBO Yogurt (e.g., to 2 tablespoons), then building up to our ½-cup serving over time. You can also take activated charcoal to bind endotoxin, 1,000 mg in capsule form, whenever these feelings occur, obtaining relief typically within 15 minutes of consumption. (Please ignore advice to use other agents, such as bentonite clay, as this is a source of toxic levels of lead.)

After eradicating SIBO, it is a good practice to continue consumption of the SIBO Yogurt two or three times per week, as this practice has proven useful in preventing the otherwise common recurrences of SIBO. You may also want to continue all the incredible benefits that accompany consumption of these microbes, especially *L. reuteri*, such as deeper sleep, greater muscle mass, smoother skin. Some people choose to simply continue the *L. reuteri* fermented alone after SIBO eradication, and that seems to work for many. You can find the recipe for fermenting SIBO Yogurt in Appendix B.

Susan, 78

"I WAS VERY ILL WITH CONTINUAL DIARRHEA, SKIN RASHES, joint pain, severe anxiety, and much more.

"By learning to make fermented dairy and other fermented foods, I boosted my health way beyond what I ever imagined. For example, *L. Reuteri* Yogurt gave me so many great benefits—it was like I took an age-reversing drug. It's not a drug but a microbe that helps boost oxytocin, which gives me a feeling of well-being. Even when I was sick with COVID, I felt positive. *L reuteri* dulls my appetite. It reduced wrinkles on my face. And that's really something because I was in the sun for years. *L reuteri* gave me a huge rush of empathy not long after I first started taking it. I felt closer to my partner and family.

"I was finally able to build muscle again like I did when I was younger. I had dysbiosis and learned how to rid myself of endotoxemia. Because of what I saw happen to my parents in their elder years, I feel so fortunate that I probably won't suffer the same horrible ailments they suffered."

BUMP AND GRIND

I hope that, by now, you are coming to appreciate that doing more of the same thing yielding short-term results followed by long-term disappointments, then blaming yourself for inadequate commitment or moral weakness, will not point you in the direction of meaningful solutions. And you should not be enticed by Hollywood celebrities boasting about how an injectable drug worked its magic on their appetite and weight—just give it time and you will see this health time bomb go off and the fireworks of tears and blame begin.

Many of the benefits of restoring lost microbes that exert dramatic effects on shape and body composition illustrate the power of the so-called gut-brain axis operating in parallel to the gut-muscle axis. If *L. reuteri* and its two friends represent just one example of these extremely powerful phenomena, what else can we restore that has been lost to the modern human experience with consequences for body shape and composition? Let's consider that next.

6

YOU DON'T KNOW WHAT
YOU'RE MISSING

YOU LIKELY DIDN'T BOIL A CARCASS TO MOBILIZE THE COLLA-
gen from cartilage, tendons, and ligaments. You don't consume
brain or skin and thereby obtain no hyaluronic acid. Anyone who
avoids animal products therefore obtains zero quantities of these body-
shaping nutrients, as they are exclusively sourced from animal organs,
meats, and other body parts. As we shall discuss, increasing your intake
of these two factors not only reduces abdominal fat and increases lean
muscle mass but also provides significant benefits for the skin, joints,
arteries, and brain. And you likely obtain little or none in your modern
version of diet created by following dietary guidelines or the advice of
most doctors and dietitians. Likewise, the modern reliance on fast food
and ultraprocessed products means that dietary intake of body-shaping
anti-inflammatory carotenoids is woefully lacking.

Ironically, most females are well aware of the benefits of collagen
and hyaluronic acid applied *topically*. I see ladies spending extraordinary sums, for instance, purchasing hyaluronic acid serums applied
to the skin. There can indeed be modest benefits from spot topical
application of this fiber. But the real benefit comes when restoring
hyaluronic acid and collagen via *oral* consumption.

Also, as previously discussed, overreliance on modern ultra-processed foods has resulted in a marked reduction in the intake of carotenoids, such as beta-carotene, lutein, zeaxanthin, and hundreds of others. Like collagen and hyaluronic acid, carotenoids also exert important effects on shape and body composition. A heaping bowl of macaroni and cheese is virtually devoid of carotenoids, as is an iceberg lettuce salad with a high-fructose corn syrup–containing low-fat salad dressing. A return to unprocessed foods, especially organic vegetables or those you've grown yourself, boosts carotenoid intake. But, because I believe that you are interested in effects that are rapid and substantial, we take advantage of the most potent carotenoid of all, astaxanthin, with body-shaping effects of its own that amplify the benefits of *L. reuteri*, collagen, and hyaluronic acid. We will dive deeper into how and why this unique carotenoid can amplify and accelerate your return to youthful body contours.

Let's explore the role of each of these factors lacking in the modern diet that, when restored, add to your ability to reshape your body contours.

COLLAGEN: PROTEIN OF LIFE AND YOUTHFULNESS

The human body, to an astonishing degree, is made of collagen. Twenty-five to 30 percent of total body protein is collagen, exceeding numerous other common proteins, such as hemoglobin, muscle proteins, and antibody proteins. You may be many things—a loving partner, parent, hardworking member of society—but you are also largely collagen. If you are a multicellular creature and not a single-celled microbe, you are packed solid with collagen. Collagen is found in every organ of the body. It is the stuff that holds you together in one piece, binding muscle, skin, bone, joints, arteries, heart, and other organs. Without this protein and its unique structural and tensile strength, you would crumble into an amorphous pile. Allow collagen proteins throughout your body to degrade, and you will age faster than you should: arthritis, skin aging, atherosclerosis, and so on, all the familiar phenomena of aging and disease.

Human organs are capable of manufacturing this essential protein. But just as your body can manufacture fat yet still requires specific fats from diet (think: dietary intake of omega-3 fatty acids, linolenic acid, linoleic acid, and oleic acid, fats that you need for survival), so it goes with collagen. Multiple cells in the body can manufacture collagen, but benefits are augmented by dietary intake. Unfortunately, modern people, given misguided dietary advice, obtain little collagen in their diets. A modest amount comes from the marbling in beef or pork: the skin, tendons, and bone in sardines; the skin on chicken wings. But a major source of collagen is organ meats. Show me someone who continues to consume organ meats, and I will show you someone who has ignored modern dietary advice.

Not only has misguided dietary advice and proliferation of processed foods caused us to abandon consumption of most collagen-rich foods, but such practices also cause *accelerated degradation* of collagen. Collagen is unusually susceptible to a chemical reaction called glycation, the glucose modification of proteins. Collagen distributed throughout the human body undergoes the process of glycation every time your blood glucose exceeds 100 mg/dl, which it does with any bite of bagel, multigrain bread, bowl of ice cream, or sips of sugary soft drink. When collagen is glycated, it becomes irreversibly brittle. In the skin, for instance, glycation leads to disorganization and breakdown of collagen proteins that accelerate dermal thinning, dryness ("crepey" skin), and increased wrinkles. In joints, glycated collagen causes cartilage in knees and hips to become brittle and break down, leading to bone-on-bone arthritis. In arteries, glycated collagen causes arteries to become rigid, increasing high blood pressure and accelerating the accumulation of atherosclerotic plaque that leads to heart attacks and sudden cardiac death. In short, glycated collagen accelerates the phenomena of aging. And it is made worse by following conventional dietary advice.[1]

Couple advice to avoid consumption of foods that would have provided collagen with the acceleration of aging and disease that develops with increased collagen glycation, and a perfect storm of aging and disease has been created.

Thankfully, even after decades of neglecting collagen intake, you have been given a second chance and can correct this fatal error. Oral ingestion of collagen also serves to replace damaged glycated collagen. Ingested collagen exerts a major influence over body shape and composition, reducing abdominal fat and increasing muscle. In one study, elderly men who engaged in a modest strength-training program for ninety days and supplemented collagen daily gained 50 percent more muscle and lost 57 percent more fat than did men who engaged in exercise alone without collagen.[2] Similar effects have been observed in studies involving younger males and females.[3,4] In other words, the body composition benefits of collagen apply regardless of age and sex and apply to anyone whose body is largely made of collagen. These benefits are unique to the collagen form of protein, with lesser benefits on body composition compared to other proteins such as whey.[5] Go ahead and add a protein supplement to your morning smoothie routine, but without collagen, you will not obtain the benefits of this unique form of protein.

For years, many expressed skepticism over whether collagen—just a protein, after all—could provide such unique effects. If you eat eggs or pork chops, both rich in protein, you will not experience a marked change in body composition or advantageous effects on skin, joints, or abdominal fat. But recent research has indeed demonstrated that collagen is unique among proteins. Like other proteins, collagen is composed of chains of amino acids. If you eat the protein of an egg, your digestive system is able to degrade egg proteins into single amino acids. If you eat a piece of pork loin or beef, you also degrade these proteins into single amino acids to supply your body with the materials needed to make body proteins. But recent evidence tells us that *collagen is different*: There are unique amino acid sequences in collagen that cannot be digested by human digestive enzymes, di- and tri-peptide (two- and three-amino acid sequences) for which no human digestive enzyme can further degrade into single amino acids. It has therefore been established that such di- and tri-peptides (such as glycine-proline-hydroxyproline, a.k.a. gly-pro-hyp) are absorbed intact and make their way to the dermal layer of skin, joint cartilage, brain, arteries, and other body sites where they amplify production of collagen in those organs, coming to the assistance of your own body's capacity for collagen production.[6] There is now more than ample evidence to show that collagen, sourced from cows (bovine), pigs (porcine), or chicken, 20 grams per day, exerts beneficial body composition effects. Collagen products are widely available and readily mix with various foods, such as yogurts, kefirs, and smoothies, or can even be used in baking. The bulk of evidence suggests that 20 grams per day is the quantity that yields maximum benefit, replacing the damaged collagen in skin and joints while also making a contribution to reshaping body contours. Later in the book, I shall provide some ideas for recipes that can be used to increase your collagen intake every day.

HYALURONIC ACID: MASTER FIBER

Over the past half century, we have been advised that increased intake of fiber is beneficial for health. Many people therefore loaded up on bran cereals and whole-grain products rich in cellulose fiber, a form of fiber that is indigestible to humans (but digestible by ruminants like goats, horses, and cows with four stomach compartments) that provide "bulk"—increased content of plant fibers in fecal material to assist its passage through the GI tract. Consume more of something that is, biochemically speaking, little different from consuming sawdust, and we were told that wonderful health effects would emerge. And perhaps there is an ounce of truth in such pronouncements. Lost in the low-fat dietary fray was a fiber that provides huge benefits, unique in that it is not sourced from grains or plants but from animals: hyaluronic acid, richest in the brain, skin, joints, eyes, and other organs that you would have consumed had you not abandoned them. As with collagen, the body is able to manufacture hyaluronic acid, but oral intake augments its body-wide benefits.

Hyaluronic acid is a polymer, a chain of molecules, not a chain of amino acids like collagen, but of sugars. Many are unaware that fibers, whether cellulose, the fiber in legumes, or hyaluronic acid, are all polymers of sugars. But they are polymers of sugars for which the human digestive system lacks the enzymes to degrade, just as we lack the enzymes to digest some of the amino acid sequences in collagen. Fiber polymers of sugars therefore do not exert all the bad effects of such sugars as sucrose (table sugar) or fructose. The direct effects of hyaluronic acid on body composition are modest, facilitating a small reduction in abdominal fat. The real magic of hyaluronic acid fiber is exerted *indirectly* through effects on microbes living in the human GI tract, serving to amplify the benefits of the gut-muscle axis. Hyaluronic acid is digested by microbes, provoking a spectacular bloom in beneficial microbial species. This, in turn, causes an increase in the production of the fatty acid butyrate, which is absorbed into our bloodstream and exerts such effects as reduction in insulin resistance, abdominal visceral fat, blood sugar, and inflammation, all factors that make their own contribution to yielding control over weight and body composition.[7] Yet again, low-fat, low-cholesterol advice deprived everyone of another crucial factor in controlling where fat is deposited and how much muscle you enjoy. Feel free to continue to enjoy the modest skin benefits of applying hyaluronic acid topically to the skin around your eyes or other surface areas, but you can amplify the benefits of this animal-sourced fiber hugely by restoring its consumption orally.

Lack of hyaluronic acid also leads to accelerated skin aging by allowing collagen loss and loss of moisture in the dermal layer. It accelerates deterioration of joint health because you lacked this important component of joint-lubricating synovial fluid. It probably also accelerates deterioration of brain health, since the brain is the most hyaluronic acid–rich organ of the body, as well as increases cardiovascular risk because arteries are meant to be lined by a protective layer of hyaluronic acid (the so-called arterial glycocalyx). Inexplicably, injecting hyaluronic acid into the face as "filler" to reduce wrinkles or into joint spaces of the knees or hips to relieve arthritis pain is a popular procedure that totally ignores the fact that hyaluronic acid can make its way to those body locations through oral ingestion.[8,9]

You could, of course, begin your journey of restoring hyaluronic acid by consuming organs rich in this factor, such as skin and brain, but I'll bet you yelled out "No way!" with that idea. So, like collagen, we supplement hyaluronic acid as a supplement powder. Most studies that demonstrate benefit have used 120 mg per day as the dose with maximum effect.

COLLAGEN AND HYALURONIC ACID: TOPICAL OR ORAL?

Apply such nutrients as collagen and hyaluronic acid to the skin around the eyes—will this yield improvements in skin on the chest, neck, or thighs? Will this provide joint, heart, arterial, and other benefits to other parts of the body? No, of course not.

This is because the outer layer of skin, the epidermis, is, by design, relatively impermeable. This is for your safety, else many everyday things we come in contact with would be absorbed into the skin, the bloodstream, and the rest of the body. Think, for instance, of laundry detergent or spray-on bathroom cleaners—we would not want such chemicals to be absorbed into our bodies. The outer skin of fish, alligators, and other creatures all share similar impermeability.

Collagen, a lengthy natural protein, and hyaluronic acid, a lengthy natural fiber, are normally present in large quantities throughout the body in all human organs. We need to obtain substantial quantities of collagen and hyaluronic acid from diet to add to the quantities of each that your body produces. Both are sourced only from animal products. (Please ignore online conversations that tell you there are plant sources of collagen and hyaluronic acid—this is simply not true. Just as liver and tongue can only originate from animals, never from lettuce or beans, likewise collagen and hyaluronic acid are strictly animal sourced.) Apply them to the skin around your eyes or other facial locations in the hopes of enjoying improved skin texture and reduction of wrinkles and you may, at best, enjoy modest improvements at the site of application—but nowhere else.

It is the dermal layer of skin, just below the relatively imper-meable external epidermis, that is the seat of skin health. It is the dermal layer where fibroblast cells produce collagen, a determinant of the depth of skin wrinkles and thereby how smooth and youthful your skin is. It is also the dermal layer where hyaluronic acid, also produced by fibroblasts, binds water molecules and thereby increases skin moisture and further stimulates collagen production that reduces wrinkle depth, the so-called plumping effect. Topical application is *local* and *superficial*, washed off with your nightly skin routine. The true determinant of skin health and appearance is therefore the dermal layer of skin, accessed through oral consumption of nutrients, not topical application.

Then, how can someone increase dermal collagen and hyaluronic acid if it fails to penetrate into the dermis with topical application? And how can you enjoy such beneficial effects, body wide, as skin improvements of the neck, chest, or thighs; improved joint health from increased collagen in cartilage and increased quantities of lubricating joint fluid; as well as shape- and body composition–modifying effects, such as reduced abdominal visceral fat and increased muscle?

Consume them orally, of course, which allows body-wide distribution of beneficial effects. After being bombarded for fifty years on the dangers of consuming saturated fat, cholesterol, and animal products, most of us now cringe at the thought of resurrecting consumption of organ meats. You'd probably rather endure a case of the flu than have a serving of stomach or tongue with a salad. Yet the evidence is clear: Collagen and hyaluronic acid are major factors in determining shape and body composition when consumed orally, as they should have been through diet all along.

Of course, you can continue your topical products, but think just how much better you'll look when you've increased dermal collagen and moisture, then apply your topical products to healthier, smoother, more youthful skin obtained from the inside out while also adding to a reduction in abdominal fat and waist circumference and restoring youthful contours of muscle from the face on down.

ASTAXANTHIN: THE ANTI-FAST FOOD NUTRIENT

Microwave a frozen food dinner and you have likely received little in the way of carotenoids. Have your meal handed to you in a paper bag at a fast-food drive-thru window and you will enjoy little carotenoid content from the burrito, burger, or fries. Have a bowl of fiber-rich bran cereal in skim milk and, once again, little to no carotenoids are in sight.

Although lacking in the modern diet for reasons distinct from why we abandoned intake of collagen and hyaluronic acid—organ meat consumption—carotenoids can yield additional benefits for health. Because dietary carotenoids are important blockers of the process of oxidative stress that causes inflammation, carotenoids are proving to be important factors in slowing the many manifestations of aging, from macular degeneration to cancer.[10]

And, of interest to our body-shape ambitions, astaxanthin, the most potent carotenoid of all, is proving to exert a major influence over abdominal fat. In one study, elderly participants given astaxanthin were able to walk longer distances independently while enjoying a 3-centimeter (1.2-inch) reduction in waist size despite no change in diet or exercise.[11] Another study corroborated the finding that exercise performance is improved with astaxanthin, but that strength and muscle mass also increased.[12] This unique carotenoid also has the ability to selectively target loss of abdominal visceral fat while also reducing many of the abnormal health phenomena associated with this fat depot and increasing levels of beneficial hormones.[13] The effects of astaxanthin alone on fat and muscle measures are impressive but we, of course, are going to amplify these effects when astaxanthin is combined with other body composition–modifying strategies. Because it is difficult, even hazardous, to obtain effective intakes of astaxanthin from such foods as salmon and shrimp, we again resort to the supplement form, 4 mg per day. We add further to restoring other carotenoids, such as lycopene, by including colorful vegetables, including the peppers and kale prominently found in the recipe section of *SUPER Body*. Even better, we will be fermenting carotenoid-rich foods to increase the bio-availability of the various carotenoids.[14]

Restore these nutrients nearly absent from the modern diet while also restoring gastrointestinal microbes lost by nearly all modern people, and you have a unique and powerful synergistic combination that can magnificently improve shape and body composition while also restoring numerous aspects of health.

It's an odd but fascinating collaboration: Combine the effects of microbes with nonmicrobial cofactors, all of which are absent or lacking from modern lifestyles, and you obtain powerful, synergistic effects. You can see that these strategies synergize in a number of ways: direct effects on muscle through oxytocin; indirect effects on reducing insulin resistance, inflammation, and the body-distorting effects of such hormones as cortisol and insulin; additional indirect effects exerted through favorable changes in the GI microbiome. We thereby witness reductions in waist circumference and all the health benefits it brings, restore youthful muscle and reverse myosteatosis, and have to give no thought to unintended adverse consequences such as regaining of weight, draining financial savings, nutrient deficiencies, SIBO, or any of the other factors that complicate conventional methods of weight loss.

BACK TO THE WILD

Most of us are unwilling to return to the ways of our ancient ancestors, killing our next meal for meat and organs, drinking from a stream or river, or submitting to ancient rituals rooted in fear and uncertainty. But can we learn from such experiences, worlds in which many of the diseases that afflict modern people occur rarely, if at all?

I believe that we can. Whether you like it or not, humans have physiologically adapted to a specific way of eating. It has nothing to do with reducing fat or cholesterol, limiting calories, or engaging in more "cardio" exercise. Returning to a world in which we do not agonize over calorie or fat intake, do not exercise to "burn" calories, but simply engage in life as it once was—that is how to take back control over weight, shape, and body composition, dietary guidelines be damned.

THREE WEEKS TO BEGIN CONQUERING YOUR LUMPS, BUMPS, AND BULGES

W E'VE EXPLORED THE WHYS AND HOWS OF ALL THAT HAS gone wrong regarding distortions of body shape and composition, and why conventional notions on how to restore the human body back to its slender and vigorous proportions do not work and, in fact, make the situation worse. Let's now decipher how we can undo the entire mess. To this end, I designed a program that can be completed over three weeks: one week to adopt the dietary program; another week to adopt the nutritional supplements to compensate for any aversion you may have to consuming brain, skin, intestines, and other animal body parts, as well as other biologically disastrous dietary practices; and another week to learn how to cultivate microbes to repopulate the GI microbiome and to play important roles in determining body shape and composition.

As I've mentioned, tracking your progress will be helpful. Because the changes that unfold with this program involve loss of fat with an increase in muscle—just following body weight does not tell the entire story. If you lose, say, 30 pounds of fat but gain 10 pounds of muscle, the scale will reflect only 20 pounds lost, underestimating the significant progress you have made. I therefore suggest you track the following measures:

- Waist circumference—Using an inexpensive cloth tape measure, measure your waist circumference at the level of your belly button and record it. We expect this measure to drop significantly in ensuing weeks and months. Three to 6 inches over the initial ninety days would be typical (more in males than females, also depending on your beginning weight, insulin resistance status, etc.). See Appendix D for the simple steps to take to ensure reliable results with your measurements.

- Total body fat—This requires a body composition (bioimpedance) scale to measure. Do not rely on measurements using calipers that are popular in gyms and among personal trainers as this is too crude a measure, reflecting only subcutaneous fat and not the more important abdominal visceral fat. Even better, some bioimpedance scales also include an abdominal visceral fat "score" that you can track as it recedes.
- Lean body mass (fat-free mass)—Also requiring a bioimpedance scale. You can track the return of youthful muscle that yields substantial advantage in metabolic health and appearance and is the key to preventing weight regain. You do not want to lose *any* muscle during any weight-loss or body-reshaping effort.

(See Appendix D for a summary of these measures, including recommended resources, such as bioimpedance body scales.)

Or you can just observe your progress in the mirror: smaller waist; reduced fat in thighs, buttocks and elsewhere; firmer arms, shoulders, and thighs; and so on, reflecting the loss of both abdominal visceral and subcutaneous fat while restoring muscle from many years earlier. You should also observe changes in your face, with fewer wrinkles, especially crow's-feet around the eyes and laugh lines around the mouth, as well as firmer facial features due to reduced inflammatory edema and increased facial musculature. For the really courageous, consider a selfie or have a friend or family member take photos at the start and at some point in the future, such as in twelve weeks' time, when substantial changes should be observable. I predict that the changes will be so profound that tears will come to your eyes when you see how far you have come.

So let's begin Week 1 with diet.

7

WEEK 1: THE DIETARY BATTLE OF THE BULGE

IF CIVILIZATION WERE TO CRUMBLE TOMORROW AND YOU WERE left to fend for yourself and your family, what would you eat? Supermarkets are empty; restaurants are shuttered; there's no Grubhub or DoorDash to deliver your food; farmers' market stalls are empty. It's every person for themselves and their families. How do you and your family eat? After the first few hunting attempts, you've exhausted the few bullets for the gun you had. You now resort to the spears, clubs, and axes that humans have used for millions of years to kill their next meal.

Most of us have never experienced the desperation of hunger. Sure, we've been hungry after ordering at a restaurant, giving the waiter or waitress a hard time because the food took more than fifteen minutes to be delivered to our table. Or the line at the local drive-thru was more than a few cars long. But I'm referring to *real* desperation, the deep hunger that comes from not having eaten for a week and not knowing whether you will be able to sate your hunger in coming days or weeks while watching your family share in the wrenching uncertainty of impending starvation, an experience shared by humans for the many thousands of generations preceding us.

The gnawing desperation of hunger causes you to instinctively resort to eating the plants around you. You uncover snails, birds' eggs, frogs, turtles, shellfish, fish. You have may been squeamish at the start in smashing the head of a snake or trapping a squirrel. But such qualms vanish as you experience deep and life-threatening lack of food. You then grab your spear, club, or ax and begin to hunt. Birds, raccoons, deer—catching and killing them with your primitive tools is not so easy. But you and your fellow hunters manage, sharing the spoils of the hunt on your return to camp. You consume the animal snout to tail, every organ included. You boil the carcass with remnants of tendons, ligaments, and whatever else remains of the animal, then toss in leaves and roots you scavenged to make soups or broths, consumed hungrily since you don't know how far into the future another such feast will follow.

In this world, there are no protuberant abdomens, no buttocks too large to fit into a chair, BMIs are typically around 20, and there is no diabetes, heart disease, acne, psoriasis, Parkinson's disease, hemorrhoids, constipation, irritable bowel syndrome, ulcerative colitis, colon cancer, and other familiar conditions that anthropologists label the "diseases of civilization." Remarkably, there is also almost no tooth decay, tooth loss, or misalignment, despite the lack of dental hygiene beyond a twig to pry the fragments of wild boar from between your teeth, observed time and again from study of indigenous hunter-gatherer populations and skulls from prior civilizations that predate the modern diet.[1-4] And, no, they did not die as young adults but lived to old age, surrounded by children and grandchildren.[5]

Shouldn't this lifestyle, followed by humans over thousands of generations to accommodate dietary needs programmed into the human genetic code, which yielded a life virtually free of all the diseases that plague modern people, including freedom from the wild excesses of weight and protuberant body parts, provide important lessons on how to eat? The handful of surviving humans still living a hunter-gatherer lifestyle, populations that have been extensively studied, have a different set of health problems, mostly injury, infections, and nematode (worm) infestations, but they are wonderfully free of the diseases and body distortions that plague us.

Let's put these critical observations to use in this first week to re-create a diet compatible with our genetic heritage. Of course, there really is no need to grab any primitive hunting weapons. Instead, we are going to mimic, as best we can, the diet that is suited to your physiology and needs. This shift in lifestyle is exceptionally powerful for losing weight, shrinking abdominal fat, and reversing numerous modern health conditions. We start this first week by focusing on diet. In Weeks 2 and 3, we will then go further and address factors lost from modern lifestyles, followed by a discussion on how to restore microbes lost from the GI microbiome, all of which yield powerful synergies in shrinking abdomens and growing muscle.

SHOPPING LIST: 50,000 BC

Obviously, there were no supermarkets fifty thousand years ago. But what if, rather than gathering and killing your food, you could shop in the prehistoric equivalent of a supermarket, clothed in your skins, unwashed and unshaved? Let's play this little game of shopping for food à la 50,000 BC as if it were a modern, well-lit supermarket, complete with a butcher, produce area, and self-serve checkout. What would you buy?

Of course, there is nothing from Nabisco, Betty Crocker, Stouffer's, or Pillsbury to steer you in the direction of processed foods. The foods you have to choose from were harvested recently: picked from the vine or dug up from the ground; animal organs and meats from game killed no later than yesterday; fish, shellfish, and reptiles caught just hours earlier. Foods that are freshly caught or harvested and consumed shortly thereafter require no preservatives. Foods that are in their raw state do not need mixing or emulsifying agents. Foods sourced from the wild contain no herbicides or pesticides, and there are no genetically modified glyphosate-laden foods among them.

Food, of course, spoils. If you and your clan went through the trouble of killing a large animal, or harvested wild plants far and wide, or waded through dark waters to spear fish as they swam by, there needs to be a way to protect the food from rotting in the days and weeks after such

great effort. Before refrigeration, there was fermentation, the preservation of foods due to naturally occurring microbes resident on the surface
or from the environment, a natural process that kept food edible and safe
for weeks to months, even years. Leaving the leg of an animal, or liver,
or tongue, covered to keep the flies away, but otherwise out in the open,
guarded by one of your clan to discourage scavengers, allowed microbes
to begin to degrade the meat, so you can slice off a piece for yourself or
your family weeks later. Or you bury fish in the sand, to be recovered
months later: malodorous but nutritious. Or vegetables submerged in
water are likewise degraded by microbes resident on their surface, dis-
couraging growth of pathogenic bacteria, fungi, and molds, leaving you
with food that is edible even deep into a cold winter or extended drought
with nutrition amplified by microbial breakdown.

Personal hygiene was, by modern standards, substandard. There
were no toilets that flushed away the remains of your last few meals, no
running water to wash your hands; sexual activity was something conducted in a cave or hut, hopefully under cover of some animal skins,
with livestock and family members just a few feet away. You therefore
do not need to look for soap, body wash, or shampoo. Because tooth
decay or other dental diseases were rare, there's no need to find tooth-
paste, dental floss, or mouthwash.

One of the toughest hurdles to overcome in rebuilding a young,
sexy, healthy body shape is to forget nearly everything you've been
told about diet. It's not easy as these misguided messages are echoed
repeatedly by media, by doctors and others who offer diet advice, by
friends and neighbors and others persuaded by the barrage of messaging from modern media. A visit to your local supermarket or big-box
store will reveal what dietary guidelines and exploitative food companies have accomplished. We are therefore going to ignore advice to
limit saturated fat, limit calorie intake, consume more "healthy whole
grains" or fiber, "move more, eat less," "everything in moderation," and
all the other familiar mantras of "healthy eating." Not only do they *not*
work, but such ideas are part of the problem.

You may gag on your cabernet, contemplating what the previous 99 percent of human life on this planet may have looked and smelled like. But, like it or not, those behaviors laid the groundwork for what your human genetics and physiology expect. There are no caramel macchiatos or Doritos Flamin' Hot Nacho Flavored Tortilla Chips here. There are no microwave ovens, no frozen preprepared dinners, no aisles and aisles of ultraprocessed pretzels, crackers, cookies, and chips. There are no ice creams, frozen yogurts, or salad dressings containing polysorbate 80 or carrageenan. There's just real, whole foods harvested from the wild to provide all the nutrition your human body needs.

So, if we were to shop the aisles of this Flintstones-style supermarket, what would we observe? We would see that:

- Nothing is packaged, freeze-dried, microwaveable, just-add-water but food is to be consumed as soon as possible unless fermented.
- Some foods are meant to be consumed raw; others require cooking over a fire.
- There are no emulsifying or mixing agents, preservatives, or artificial colors or flavors added.
- Nothing contains grains (as wheat, corn, and grains are recent additions, added many tens of thousands of years later after our 50,000 BC visit).
- There are no highly processed oils, such as corn, canola, grapeseed, cottonseed, or "mixed vegetable" oil; only lard, tallow, the fats from meats and organs, and (if a tropical climate) coconut and palm.
- The only sources of sugar are wild, fiber-rich fruit, entirely unlike modern fruit, and the occasional honeycomb containing honey stolen from bees.
- There is a special fermented food section with fermented vegetables, fruit, meats, and organs, naturally preserving flavors and improving nutritional value.

You cannot, of course, travel back over five hundred centuries to shop in such an imaginary store. But your genetic code and physiology are assuming that you are, indeed, shopping in a store of wild, fresh, whole foods.

In your local modern supermarket, are there any wild plants and roots? Very few, if any. Birds' eggs, rich in the nutrients obtained from consumption of worms and insects? No, but you'll find eggs coming from large warehouse-like operations in which thousands of chickens are fed corn, antibiotics, and other synthetic ingredients designed to yield volume, not nutrients. Meat and organs obtained from animals allowed to graze freely on grasses and forage, rich in fats, linolenic acid, various other nutrients, absent growth hormone and antibiotics— look hard and long for such products in a modern store.

Viewed from the perspective of all that has gone wrong in diet due to misguided dietary guidelines and the proliferation of processed foods, it should come as no surprise that, as a species, we are experiencing an unprecedented degree of distortions of health and body shape and composition. We have defied the wisdom built into our genetic code. Living a modern life, we have, as a society, been hoping to obtain dietary needs through foods wrapped in cellophane or in microwave-safe trays—but the experiment has been a failure.

The shopping list of 50,000 BC is therefore quite different from the shopping list of our time. In our world, we shop for bargains, foods to please friends at the Sunday football gathering or children whooping it up at the seven-year-old's birthday party. In our modern world, we may have sanitary sewage and running water, but we have lost touch with what it is we, as members of the species *Homo sapiens*, should be hunting and gathering.

Can we reestablish a connection to our prehistoric selves, experiencing freedom from modern diseases while enjoying flat abdomens, muscular and sinew-laden arms and legs, vigor and agility maintained up to our tenth decade? I believe that it is indeed possible, even readily attainable. I'd like you to picture yourself as a hungry, loincloth-clad member of a clan of humans, hunting and foraging for foods to feed yourself and your family, carving out a life on this planet minus all the ads, billboards, discounts, and tempting tastes of ultraprocessed foods. You will likely not kill any creature today, nor will you gather nuts or berries or dig in the forest for roots. But let's just pretend that you will so that you are able to tap into your inner wild, instinctively eating *Homo sapiens*.

DIETARY DRAMA

It's been a uniquely twenty-first-century phenomenon: the proliferation of documentary dramas that purport to teach us how to eat.

Of course, had dietary guidelines and dietary "authorities" got it right from the start, there would be no need for such media productions, nor would there be a need for someone like me to suggest how you should think about diet. While it is always a good thing to stimulate conversation about something so fundamental and important to health as nutrition, it also allows plenty of misinterpretation, misrepresentation, and for various groups to advance their own agendas. It could be veganism or vegetarianism, or ketogenic or "Paleo" dieting; it could be something as outrageous as being a "frugivore" (surviving strictly on fruit) or engaging in the baby food or grapefruit diets, real diets embraced by millions of people.

A recent production that gained a lot of attention detailed a study labeled the "Stanford Twin Study" in which twenty-two identical twin pairs participated, one member of a twin pair assigned to a vegan diet, the other to a "healthy" omnivorous diet.[6] Over eight weeks, the vegan participants experienced modestly lower LDL cholesterol, fasting insulin, and a blood compound called trimethylamine oxide (TMAO), a marker purported to add to cardiovascular risk. The findings of the study have been broadly advertised as the Netflix documentary *You Are What You Eat*, with the vegan/vegetarian communities hailing the findings of the study as finally validating what they have been arguing for years: that a vegan or vegetarian lifestyle is healthier.

Is this true? Let's take a closer look at the findings. Pull back the curtain and you will find that numerous errors and misinterpretations were committed that led to false conclusions. Among them:

- Vegans experienced a 15-mg/dl reduction in LDL cholesterol, while omnivores experienced no change. Brushed aside was a reduction in HDL cholesterol and rise in triglycerides in vegan participants. In other words, observations were based on an antiquated method of gauging cardiovascular risk, one that includes a calculation (not measurement) of LDL cholesterol, a calculation that is invalidated by any significant change in diet and thereby no longer reflects reality. The drop in HDL and rise in triglycerides, however, suggest that, had a superior method of advanced lipoprotein testing been applied (e.g., nuclear magnetic resonance [NMR] testing that quantifies and characterizes the particles that actually cause heart disease), there would have been an increase in very low-density lipoproteins (VLDL) and small LDL particles (both driven by increased triglyceride availability), the real causes of coronary heart disease.[7] In short, an outdated method yielded the direct opposite of what likely really happened: *increased* cardiovascular risk in vegan participants.

- Intake of vitamin B_{12} and iron dropped among the vegan participants, though no overt deficiency developed over the eight weeks of the study. But we already know with confidence from other studies that, over a longer time period, deficiencies of both B_{12} and iron develop with high frequency, along with deficiencies of zinc, omega-3 fatty acids, collagen, and hyaluronic acid.[8] If you need to supplement half a dozen nutrients to compensate for the deficiencies of diet, then the problem is the diet. (The nutritional supplements that are included in the lifestyle discussed in *SUPER Body* are not intended to compensate for the deficiencies of the diet, but *deficiencies of modern lifestyles*, such as relying on filtered drinking water, not obtaining sufficient sun exposure, and avoiding consumption of organ meats.)

If veganism is coupled with inclusion of grains, then mineral deficiencies can also develop or worsen due to the presence of grain phytates that bind magnesium, iron, zinc, and calcium and make them unavailable for absorption.

- Dietary intake of cholesterol dropped dramatically in vegans compared to no change in omnivores. However, the notion that dietary cholesterol increases risk for heart disease has been debunked over the past three decades and no one continues to advocate reducing dietary cholesterol.[9] This is just window dressing.

- The purported cardiovascular risk marker, TMAO, dropped modestly among vegans with no change in omnivores. The fundamental error made in this, as well as the original study suggesting that increased TMAO from consumption of animal products increases cardiovascular risk, is that the GI microbiome is regarded as a black box, ignoring the fact that undesirable increases in specific bacterial species are the driver of TMAO, not food. In other words, the input (food) is not the primary driver of TMAO production; it's the composition of the GI microbiome that is disrupted and thereby can yield greater quantities of TMAO.[10] Vegan participants included greater consumption of fibers from vegetables and legumes compared to negligible intake in omnivores, thereby likely experiencing favorable changes in GI microbiome composition that yielded less TMAO. The issue was likely not the lack of animal-sourced foods in vegans but the lack of fibers from vegetables and legumes in the omnivores, an issue easily remedied by inclusion of vegetables and legumes.

The widely publicized Stanford Twin Study is therefore an effort based on tracking flawed, outdated biomarkers—failure to factor in the contribution of fiber intake and changes in microbiome composition—but with findings that suit the agenda of a certain segment of the eating public and some documentary filmmakers. Had better biomarkers been tracked, it is likely that the vegan diet would have been exposed as inferior. If the differences boil down to fiber intake, not animal products, the remedy for the omnivorous diet, or for any diet for that matter, is to simply include fibers that nourish microbes, regardless of the presence or absence of meats.

It is worth noting that satisfaction with diet plummeted among vegan participants while remaining unchanged in omnivores. This is understandable because a vegan diet is counter to the evolutionary, adaptive dietary experience of our species. Of course, we do not have to subscribe to one or the other diet, but create a diet that draws from the advantages of both: greater dietary satisfaction with inclusion of animal products; the inclusion of collagen and hyaluronic acid sources; increased intake of plant matter and legumes for microbiome effects; exclusion of wheat, grains, and sugar to eliminate all their harmful effects. You can appreciate that posing a dietary dichotomy of vegan versus omnivorous diet is a fatal oversimplification that, unfortunately, does not stop headlines from broadcasting faulty conclusions.

"SALE ON PIG'S KNUCKLES IN AISLE 7"

Is it even possible to re-create the diet of 50,000 BC, given the choices we have among modern foods? It is, though not perfectly. Unfortunately, we cannot avoid the ubiquitous herbicide glyphosate, since it has been so widely overused that it even contaminates organic food.[11] Order a meal at a nice restaurant, and your steak or salmon was likely seared in corn or canola oil in nonstick cookware leaching out unhealthy chemicals (e.g., polyfluorinated substances [PFAS]). A beautifully prepared salad at an upscale steak house is likely contaminated by multiple herbicides and pesticides that lace the lettuce, onions, and shredded carrots, not to mention the high-fructose corn syrup, sugar, and polysorbate 80 in the ranch or Italian dressing.

We have to be realistic. Just as we are not about to club a bear on the snout, or harvest wild roots and mushrooms from the forest or jungle, we have to pick and choose from the shrinking list of real, whole foods that are still available to us. It also means that we need to cover our eyes and plug our ears to the barrage of marketing that comes our way through media, telling us to get more fiber from bran cereals, or that we can eat "fresh" at the local drive-thru window, or that a diet low in animal products and weighed more heavily in favor of fruits and vegetables obviates all the problems associated with modern foods—none of this is true.

Short of growing all your own food or hunting your own sources of meats and organs, how can you conduct your life yet remain true to your dietary genetic heritage? Let's be clear: It's not that easy. There is great profit in persuading you that eating snack chips coated with spices is perfectly acceptable, or that microwaveable pizza is a source of healthy vegetables—billions of dollars annually are at stake in keeping you coming back for such processed foods. After all, if you purchase a few organic peppers from the local farmers' market or, heaven forbid, grow lettuce and eggplant in your backyard garden, how do multibillion-dollar food conglomerates profit from the process? They do not.

So recognize that Big Agribusiness and Big Food are, for the most part, out for profit and their products have little or nothing to do with health, despite claims of "low in fat" or "rich in fiber" or "with added vitamin C."

Therefore, let's develop a dietary code of behavior that mimics, as best we can in today's industrialized food world, the dietary habits of someone from fifty thousand years ago. While it may not be as easy as just ordering food from Amazon, or pulling up to the drive-thru window at Arby's, it should be easier than it was in 50,000 BC, since there is no need to dig or hunt, and you do indeed have the conveniences provided by refrigeration and indoor plumbing.

DIET AND CONTROL OVER SHAPE AND BODY COMPOSITION

To make this dietary approach manageable, I am going to provide guidelines to help you, as best you can, re-create the diet of our ancestors, the diet programmed into the human genetic code to serve your basic physiologic needs. You will find no advertisements or dietary guidelines here, only cool logic aimed at unmasking the prehistoric human hidden inside you, aching to escape the protuberant abdomen, ectopic fat, lost muscle, and other health and body distortions acquired by living your modern life.

What may be notable in these guidelines is what is *not* here: There is no calorie counting, no advice to "move more, eat less," no limiting fat or saturated fat or cholesterol, no "eat more healthy whole grains," or other popular mantras of nutrition that, despite evidence to the contrary, still prevail.

There are, undoubtedly, hurdles beyond clearing your brain of the barrage of misinformation of the past. Let's therefore discuss some of the "ground rules" that I have distilled down to eight steps to build a nutritional foundation for your body shape–modifying program. Each of these eight basic strategies stacks the odds in favor of generating healthy, youthful body contours:

1. Choose whole, unprocessed foods.
2. Choose organic foods whenever possible.
3. Avoid all wheat and other grain products.
4. Avoid gluten-free processed foods.
5. Never limit calories.
6. Never limit fat or oil intake.
7. Avoid added sugar.
8. Drink filtered water.

Some of these strategies may already be familiar to you, but now we fold in a few additional strategies that amplify your hopes of reachieving desirable body contours.

So, here we go, a dietary back-to-the-wild approach for modern people to gain control over shape and body composition as well as health:

Choose whole, unprocessed foods—An egg, avocado, slice of pork or beef would qualify as unprocessed; these are foods minimally altered or unaltered by modern food processing. Meats, poultry, fish, and eggs are easier to recognize as unprocessed, but be sure to avoid lean cuts, low-fat ground meats, rotisserie or other preprepared poultry, fish cakes, chicken fingers, and so on. They should be as close to their original butchered or captured form as possible. You sacrifice convenience, yes, but you gain control over the quality and contents of your food. This is how we avoid preservatives, food colorings, emulsifying agents, and other health-damaging additives. Meats from pastured animals, rather than a concentrated animal-feeding operation confining thousands of animals in cramped spaces, improve nutritional value even further. Take this one initial step of returning to whole, unprocessed foods and you have avoided a long list of unhealthy modern food components.

We thereby minimize exposure to preservatives (e.g., potassium sorbate, sodium benzoate, nitrites, butylated hydroxy anisol [BHA], butylated hydroxyl toluene [BHT], and many others), emulsifying agents (e.g., carboxymethylcellulose, polysorbate 80, carrageenan), synthetic sweeteners (aspartame, sucralose, saccharine) that exert destructive effects on bowel flora composition, flour-whitening agents (e.g., azodicarbonamide, titanium dioxide), and processed oils (e.g., corn oil, "vegetable" oil, hydrogenated oil, grapeseed oil, cottonseed oil, canola oil).[12,13]

Choose organic—whenever possible, especially if the exterior will be consumed. For example, strawberries or blueberries that you consume whole should always be organic, but a tangerine whose peel you discard is not so important to consume organic. Lentils, beans, and peas will be consumed whole, of course, so make them organic. Ideally, grow as much as you can yourself, since you are not going to spray your garden with glyphosate or other herbicides. We therefore include plenty of organic lettuces, kale, spinach, leeks, dandelion greens, broccoli, and other vegetables. Try to make your coffees and teas organic, as conventionally raised coffee beans and leaves of the *Camellia sinensis* tea plant are often heavily sprayed with herbicides and pesticides.

There are plenty of reasons to make your food choices organic. This is a designation that would not have been necessary if traditional farming methods were still being applied, such as use of organic fertilizers, cultivating a variety of foods and not the modern practice of monoculture (e.g., huge fields of genetically modified corn or soy). It's sobering to recall that Rachel Carson's book *Silent Spring* sounded the alarm on excessive reliance on synthetic pesticides and herbicides over sixty years ago, yet the problems stemming from modern agricultural practices have only expanded since then. The push toward high-volume production has promoted the adoption of many unhealthy agricultural practices, leaving small independent family farms behind. Herbicides and pesticides used in large-scale agricultural production act as antibiotics, endocrine disruptive factors, neurotoxins, and carcinogens upon human consumption, even in very small quantities.[14] Choosing organic, for instance, reduces your exposure to the herbicide rotenone, which has been associated with Parkinson's disease, or lindane, associated with non-Hodgkin's lymphoma. You also avoid genetically modified (GM) foods laced with glyphosate, since most GM foods are resistant to this herbicide, allowing a farmer to spray his field with it, killing weeds but not the corn, soy, or other GM crop. Thankfully, despite the critics who cite organic farming as inefficient, booming consumer demand for organic foods is driving growth of this industry, now $80 billion annually in the United States. Although there has been some public skepticism over whether foods labeled "organic" truly are, repeated analyses have demonstrated that only conventionally raised produce and meats contain significant residues of herbicides and pesticides, with minor residues in organic foods.[15] There is even a growing awareness that, like humans, soil has a microbiome. The microbial composition of soil in high-volume commercial farming creates a soil depleted of healthy microbes and nutrients, while organic methods tend to cultivate a healthy soil microbiome that also increases the nutritive value of foods, richer in vitamins, minerals, polyphenols, carotenoids, linolenic acid, and other nutrients.

Choosing whole, unprocessed, organic foods therefore minimizes the microbiome/hormonal/metabolic disruptions of farming chemicals and food additives. Big Agribusiness conglomerates won't like it, but your body will celebrate its freedom from these disruptive factors by contributing to your flat abdomen and muscled shoulders and limbs.

But because organic farming is still overpowered by foods coming from large-scale industrial farms, organic choices represent no more than 5 percent of the total, meaning you shall have to actively seek out less common organic choices.

Organic animal products also tend to come from farms that have adopted more humane practices, allowing animals to pasture, consume their natural foods, such as grass, forage, and insects, and not be confined in huge warehouses that allow no freedom of movement while being fed low-quality feed as well as antibiotics to treat rapidly communicated infectious diseases and to accelerate growth.[15]

Another reason to choose organic foods that will prove useful further in the program is that you simply cannot have herbicides, pesticides, wax coatings, or other substances on the surface of, say, cucumbers or zucchini or tomatoes that you are going to ferment, a big first step in regaining control over your gastrointestinal microbiome we'll discuss in Chapter 9.

Avoid all wheat and other grain products—Here is where we depart even more dramatically from the conventional message. Contrary to popular opinion, wheat and other grains (rye, barley, millet, rice, oats, sorghum, triticale, einkorn, emmer, spelt) are recent additions to the human diet. Banishing them from your lifestyle can yield breathtaking changes. If the time of our species on planet Earth were compressed into twenty-four hours of a clock, we added grains after 11:55 p.m., at the tail end of a long day. Wheat and grains should have never been adopted into the human diet for a long list of reasons: The gliadin protein yields an opioid appetite stimulant effect that impairs your ability to control eating habits; the carbohydrate amylopectin A has greater potential to raise blood sugar than table sugar; wheat germ agglutinin is a potent bowel toxin; and phytates bind minerals, such as iron and magnesium, causing you to pass them into the toilet—in short, the effects of wheat and grains mean you eat more food than you need, experience high blood sugar and its abdominal fat–expanding effects, and endure bowel struggles and nutrient deficiencies—a snapshot of the modern American advised to consume more "healthy whole grains."

The increases in food intake and blood sugar are major players in causing distortions of body shape, especially expansion of abdominal fat. (If you'd like an extended discussion of the rationale and evidence behind this approach, see my *Wheat Belly* books that chronicle how geneticists and agribusiness altered something initially inappropriate for human consumption, then made it worse through genetic manipulations to create what is now passed off to you as wheat and grains. Sure, there are manipulations that make it smell and taste good, but they also damage health and body composition. It is a horror story of gripping proportions—that's why I label them "Frankengrains.")

But is a grain-free lifestyle really possible, given the ubiquity of these foods in supermarkets, cafeterias, restaurants, and the eating habits of the public? It absolutely is. Yes, it means ignoring the barrage of advertisements, urgings of dietary "authorities" and most doctors, and friends and family who say things like "Just one won't hurt!"

Of course, the majority of wheat- and grain-based foods are highly processed by necessity. No one can eat wheat seeds, for instance, harvested directly from a wheat stalk. We therefore banish all breads, bagels, doughnuts, breakfast cereals, crackers, cookies, pretzels, baking mixes, cakes, pies, pasta—all the foods that have come to dominate the modern diet. We also avoid processed foods that include a wheat/grain ingredient, such as gluten, cornstarch, corn syrup, and rice and oat "milks." Consistent with choosing whole, unprocessed foods, you will find that nearly all the processed foods that typically occupy most of the inner aisles of supermarkets are off-limits.

WHERE THERE'S AN OPIATE, THERE'S ADDICTION

And where there's addiction, there's withdrawal that follows when the opiate is stopped. It happens with OxyContin, it happens with heroin, and it happens with gliadin-derived opioid peptides from wheat and related grains.[16,17] (From here on in, when I say "wheat," I am referring to *all* grains that are, after all, closely related, genetically speaking.) There may be no fentanyl-laced pretzels or crackers, but the effects of opioids originating from wheat and grains have their own collection of addictive, behavior-modifying effects.

Despite the ubiquity of wheat, humans do not have the digestive enzymes to degrade wheat proteins, such as gliadin, to single amino acids as we do when we eat an egg or piece of beef. The gliadin protein is degraded down to four or five amino acid–long peptide fragments that possess unique properties. Among their effects: crossing into the brain to bind to opioid receptors, where they trigger behavioral outbursts in children with autism and attention deficit hyperactivity disorder (ADHD), hallucinations in people with paranoid schizophrenia, depression and suicidal ideation in people with tendencies toward these conditions, food obsessions in people with bulimia and binge-eating disorder, and appetite stimulation in the rest of us.[16–21]

When people banish all wheat from their diet, about half experience a mild opiate-withdrawal syndrome characterized by fatigue, depression, nausea, and headache, phenomena that typically last three to five days, occasionally longer. (It wasn't uncommon in my cardiology practice for someone to break down and sob in the exam room, knowing that avoiding all wheat and grains would bring on unpleasant physical and emotional symptoms.) At the end of the withdrawal process, people report that they sometimes experience a feeling of euphoria, as well as release from uncontrolled appetite. But I won't kid you: The initial process can be unpleasant. To minimize the unpleasantness over these several days, consider:

- Hydrating more than usual
- Lightly salting food and water (to compensate for sodium loss in urine that occurs during this process that reduces the sodium-retaining properties of insulin resistance)
- Initiating magnesium supplementation (discussed in Chapter 8), especially if muscle cramps develop
- Pampering yourself—watch a funny movie, get a massage, call a friend

Know that the process is temporary and better days are ahead. Just as a cigarette smoker must endure the nicotine withdrawal process, wheat consumers need to get through the unpleasant business of opiate withdrawal in order to start anew with restored control over appetite, one of the cornerstones of your effort to reshape your body.

Avoid gluten-free processed foods—This confuses people after being told that we should banish all wheat and grains. But just because something is labeled "gluten-free," meaning free of the protein gluten, does not necessarily make it healthy. In fact, gluten-free processed foods, such as bagels, pasta, breads, and baking mixes are incredibly destructive to health. They are ultraprocessed, and because they are usually made with such ingredients as cornstarch, rice flour, potato starch, and tapioca starch, they raise blood sugars to the highest levels of any food (even higher than the amylopectin A of wheat and grains) and thereby cause dramatic weight gain, especially in the abdomen. They are also flagrant triggers for the formation of small LDL particles I discussed earlier that are the real cause of coronary heart disease. So we absolutely avoid such products. An avocado or an egg can be naturally gluten-free, but gluten-free processed and ultraprocessed foods should never cross your lips. After *Wheat Belly* was published, it was not uncommon that someone would claim to have read the book and come up to me and declare, "Hey, I did the *Wheat Belly* diet and gained 30 pounds and became a type 2 diabetic! Why?!" I'd ask them if they consumed gluten-free foods. "Yes, of course. Isn't that what *Wheat Belly* was about?" They would inevitably admit to skimming through the book, or relying on a friend or neighbor to provide the CliffsNotes version, neglecting to tell them to avoid gluten-free processed foods. Let's be absolutely clear: Gluten-free processed foods are awful for health, including making a major contribution to sustaining undesirable lumps, bumps, and bulges.

Never limit calories—Skipping a meal because you are not hungry or pushing away the plate of something you don't like is harmless. But never adopt a program in which you reduce calorie intake for any extended period of time. Sure, you can reduce calories for a few days, but the longer you engage in any form of calorie restriction, the more you risk loss of muscle, a reduction in metabolic rate, and triggering appetite hormones, phenomena that can last for years, ensuring weight regain *even if a low calorie intake is maintained.* I cringe to think how much money is spent for weight-loss programs, smartphone apps, pharmaceuticals, and bariatric procedures that provide methods to reduce calories that only result in temporary success but long-term weight regain or other health disasters. It's a well-charted path that has been proven ineffective but continues to stymie millions of people, including doctors.

Also be aware that fasting for more than a couple of days, a practice that has become quite popular, causes loss of muscle, just as any other method of reduced-calorie intake. In one recent study, for example, men fasted for ten days and lost around 8 pounds of muscle, and when they ended the fast, they regained more abdominal fat than when they started.[22] The brief fasts that some people practice as so-called time-restricted eating, in which the eating "window" is confined to something like eight hours, does not seem to be associated with muscle loss, however.[23] (But please do not interpret this to mean that I am endorsing time-restricted eating; I am just making the point that the brief fasts of this eating pattern don't provoke the same loss of muscle that extended fasting does.)

Follow a few simple, commonsense rules for eating: Eat when you're hungry, not according to a strict schedule. Eat until you are satisfied. Overeating is a struggle of the past, since you are not limiting fats and oils that are satiating, you have removed gliadin-derived opioid appetite stimulants, and you have the additional advantage of oxytocin that eradicates the desire to snack. You naturally and effortlessly eat what you require for survival and life performance, no more, no less. In my experience, most of the people following these ideas eat a late breakfast, then a second meal late afternoon and that's it—no need for regularly scheduled lunches or dinners.

Cutting calories is also miserable, typically generating around-the-clock food obsessions, counting the minutes until your next meal, enviously eyeing other people as they eat. None of this is necessary as you will be eating to serve your physical needs, not in response to unnatural appetite stimulants. Imagine that: eating only what you require to serve normal physiological needs. It means that you are the one least likely to find a bargain at the all-you-can-eat food buffet, as you will find that your needs represent a fraction of what others consume.

AN END TO APPETITE

The strategies advocated here result in a dramatic reduction in appetite, freeing you from the tyranny of food temptation. You will likely find yourself satisfied for extended periods, not having your day plagued by thoughts of food. You will not be tempted when walking past the box of doughnuts someone brought to the office or the scent of Cinnabon as you stroll past the shop in the mall. You are freed from appetite and temptation because:

- You eliminated gliadin protein-derived opioid peptides— Elimination of wheat and grains removed the potent opioid appetite stimulants that come from partial digestion of the gliadin protein of wheat, the secalin protein of rye, the hordein of barley, the zein of corn. Don't underestimate this effect: Just watch the grain-consuming people around you, elbowing their way to the all-you-can-eat food bar, or nervously anticipating their order at the drive-thru window while battling insatiable hunger, or impatient customers at the restaurant who find the few minutes' wait for their order intolerable. You will be freed from the effects of insatiable hunger that leads to poor food choices, effortlessly and painlessly coasting through your day with barely a thought of food. Have breakfast, for instance, of two fried eggs, sausage, and a few sips of kefir or other fermented food, and you likely won't be interested in food until two p.m., three p.m., or later. You may even forget to have lunch. Or if you have lunch, you will likely desire only a couple of bites of something for dinner. The rules are completely changed, appetite something you barely notice or think about. (You can witness this in its most extreme form in people suffering from bulimia or binge-eating disorder, people racked by 24/7 food obsessions, with obsessions dissolving completely with avoidance of all sources of the gliadin protein.) If you are a fan of this recent popular notion of time-restricted eating, these effects make it much easier. (Because our basic efforts in SUPER Body yield such powerful effects, I believe that the claims made with such efforts—living longer, weight loss, metabolic health—are overblown, particularly in the context of the efforts made here. But I don't believe that such efforts are harmful.)

- You do not limit fat and oil intake—Have more eggs, have more bacon and sausage, use more butter, include more extra-virgin olive oil in your dishes, cook with coconut oil, never trim the fat off beef, pork, or other meat. Fat not only makes food taste better, it is also satiating, leaving you satisfied for extended periods. And, no, naturally occurring, unprocessed fats and oils do not add to risk for heart disease, a common misinterpretation of the evidence. If your great-grandmother could make an appearance at your dinner table, she would grin with pride at the fatty meats, butter, and green beans sautéed in bacon fat that you serve.

- You experience a boost in oxytocin triggered by restoring the lost gut microbe *Lactobacillus reuteri*, which reduces appetite further, specifically eliminating snacking that does not serve physiologic need.[24] Think of it: The boost in oxytocin intensifies affection you have for those close to you, increases sexual desire, restores youthful characteristics, and causes you to turn away food—it's like being in love again.

Put it all together and you experience magnificent control over eating habits. You will no longer be the unwitting victim of the food industry, causing you to purchase more products regardless of the health and body-shape consequences. You will be miraculously freed of the effects of processed foods, no longer victim to the predatory practices of food conglomerates, no longer at the mercy of misinformation from doctors and other health-care practitioners.

There's a small downside: Once your eyes have been opened to the crimes against humanity being conducted under the guise of dietary guidelines and weight loss, you will be horrified at the eating behavior of the people around you who do not engage in these strategies, wolfing down huge quantities of food, angry if food is not immediately available, while suffering expanding abdominal fat and losing muscle. It is admittedly difficult to educate these people, having been so brainwashed by the popular message and unable to resist temptation. They can even get angry when you try to educate them. So don't waste your breath, but just set the example of magnificent health and slenderness and let them, over time, ask why you look so slender, muscular, and youthful. That will be your cue that it's time to share your knowledge.

Erica, 56

"I was in a desperate place when I discovered Dr. Davis. I had daily headaches, stiff and painful joints, overnight leg cramps, poor sleep and massive food intolerances. Oh, and the bloating! My diet was limited to meat, eggs, fish, some vegetables and small amounts of berries. I could no longer tolerate foods like legumes, nuts, onions, garlic, broccoli, kale, tomatoes, to name a few.

"A gut test confirmed my suspicions of leaky gut and dysbiosis. Sadly, the suggested probiotic only exacerbated symptoms. Then I stumbled upon Dr. Davis in a podcast interview and knew I was onto something different. I wasted no time in buying the AIRE device. The results from the AIRE device were as grim as the gut test. Well, what's a girl to do but make SIBO yogurt? After consuming it for just two days, bloating and other symptoms already began to diminish. Could the yogurt work that quickly? Was it just a placebo effect? No, it couldn't be because even the AIRE device began to show positive results! This was the SIBO yogurt effect!

"I am thrilled to report the following results:

I can once again eat nuts, leeks, garlic and a myriad of other foods without dreadful consequences.

That dry, red patch above my lip is gone!

I sleep so much more soundly and actually have dreams I remember!

Headaches and stiff joints upon awakening are a rarity now.

My hair stylist and I both noticed that my hair seems healthier.

My fingernails grow more quickly.

Not sure if this is too much information, but my stools don't float anymore!

"What a blessing it is to no longer feel like I'm on a downhill slide towards chronic disease."

———

Never limit fats or oils—While we avoid modern processed oils, such as corn, canola, soybean, safflower, sunflower, cottonseed, and grapeseed (that risk stoking inflammatory pathways via excess omega-6 or linoleic acid consumption), we do not limit our overall intake of fats or oils. If you have a rib eye steak, for instance, don't trim off the fat—eat it. If you have baked salmon or chicken, eat the skin, eat the dark meat, save the fat retrieved from cooking meats or poultry. Use plenty of extra-virgin olive oil, butter, and the fat you saved after making bacon.

We shall conduct ourselves much like our great-grandparents and the thousands of generations of humans that preceded them. We consume what organs we are willing to consume, and never trim the fat off meat, and *never* purchase any product labeled "low-fat" or "nonfat" or "extra-lean." Opt for full-fat dairy products, never buy lean ground meat, never buy boneless, skinless chicken breast. Enjoy bacon, ribs, and other fatty cuts of meat and then take a thick black marker and cross out the total and LDL cholesterol values on your cholesterol panel.

Avoid added sugar—You will find that after the elimination of wheat and grains, your sensitivity to sweetness in foods is amplified. Foods that were previously not sweet will now taste sweet, often sickeningly sweet. You will find, for instance, that milk chocolate and ice cream are overwhelmingly sweet, virtually inedible. Avoiding foods that have added sugar is therefore a lot easier than it sounds in the context of having eliminated wheat and grains and enjoying the satiating effect of not limiting fats and oils.

Just by banishing all wheat and grains, you have made a major dent in your intake of carbohydrates that expand abdominal fat, cause fat infiltration of muscle, and add to risk for numerous common chronic diseases. But you take it an important step further by avoiding foods with added sugars. It means avoiding obvious sources of sugar, such as candies, pastries, soft drinks, and juices. It can also mean avoiding processed foods that have sugar as an additive; these include ice cream, sauces (marinara, barbecue, teriyaki), ketchup, salad dressings, pickles, processed meats, commercial yogurts, and thousands of other products that pack the shelves of your local supermarket. If it's a processed product, it likely has added sugar—plain and simple.

Be aware that food manufacturers have been very clever in concealing the addition of sugar to their products by assigning new names to them, such as "coconut sugar" or "corn sugar" or "natural sweetener." While the names may change, the physiological consequences remain the same: All these sweeteners contribute to risk for heart disease, type 2 diabetes, and dementia, and they also expand abdominal fat, increase deposition of ectopic fat, and cause fat infiltration of muscle, ruining your hopes of regaining a youthful shape and body composition.

Unfortunately, fruit has become a challenge, as modern fruit has been cultivated and hybridized for reduced fiber and increased sugar content to please the modern sweet tooth. I think about the tart grapes I used to pick in my backyard sixty years ago, or the small sour apples that dropped from apple trees, a far cry away from today's excessively sugary seedless grapes or the huge sweet apples now sold in grocery stores. Because most of us no longer have access to wild fruit, it means picking and choosing your fruit for the least sugar content.

I therefore recommend that we follow a simple rule: Limit your exposure to no more than 15 grams net carbs per meal, "net carbs" referring to total carbohydrates minus fiber (since fiber is listed on nutritional panels as a carbohydrate, even though it is not metabolizable by human digestive enzymes). Look up the nutritional content of foods in various smartphone apps, websites, or handbooks (listed in Appendix A), and you will find that a medium-size ripe banana, for example, contains 27 grams total carbohydrates, 3 grams fiber: 27 – 3 = 24 grams net carbs—too much for your health and body remolding purposes. Half the banana would fit, provided you do not add additional carbs from other foods. By adhering to this limit, you will avoid provoking significant rises in blood insulin that would have otherwise added to expansion of abdominal fat.

This 15-gram net carb limit helps you navigate other foods safely and effectively. For instance, it also means that such foods as dried fruit (raisins, prunes, apricots, dates, cranberries, etc.) are off-limits, as they are highly concentrated in sugar content and quickly booby-trap your efforts. For example, 1 cup of dried cranberries contains 92 grams net carbs—wildly beyond our cutoff. Likewise, fruit drinks and fruit juices, cooked potatoes (all varieties), desserts, and grain-like foods, such as quinoa and buckwheat, are not worth bothering with as you will easily exceed this limit. (Later, I will show you how to make delightful effervescent juices in which the sugar is fermented out by microbes, yielding such things as mango or pomegranate soda, all with minimal carbs.) As discussed earlier, gluten-free processed foods are, ironically, among the most hazardous of all as they exceed our net carb limit, even in small portions. Further, finely pulverized gluten-free flours increase surface area for digestion and thereby raise blood sugar and insulin higher than all other foods, ensuring that you will expand abdominal fat, not to mention send blood sugar through the roof and add to your risk for heart disease, type 2 diabetes, and dementia. We therefore avoid gluten-free processed foods completely.

By following this simple net carb rule, you will find that berries are among the safest. Raspberries, blueberries, strawberries, cranberries, and other berries pack the most nutrient density for the least exposure of sugar. Serving sizes of up to ½ cup therefore remain below our 15-gram net carb cutoff. Apples, pears, citrus fruits, and others share the same issue of having been bred for low fiber and high sugar content. It is, unfortunately, easy to consume fruit in excessive quantities, given the greater sugar content of modern varieties. We therefore navigate these fruits by following our net carb rule. Another way to ensure that you stay within these limits for maximum body-shaping advantage is to follow what I call the blood glucose "No Change Rule" (see box).

THE BLOOD GLUCOSE "NO CHANGE RULE"

Here is a simple strategy that has served my community well: By ensuring no rise in blood glucose with a meal, you accelerate weight loss from abdominal fat while also allowing greater control over blood sugars and insulin. Although I describe this concept to help you gain faster and more complete control over shape and body composition, the same rule can also be used to reverse type 2 diabetes—yes, the same device used to manage the disease can also be used to get rid of the disease, even if doctors don't tell you this. (However, if you have been prescribed blood sugar–reducing medication, such as metformin or insulin, it is best to work with your doctor to help you reduce, then eliminate these medications to prevent any episodes of hypoglycemia [low blood glucose]. If your doctor refuses to work with you, find one that will—it's that important.)

You will need a glucose meter, test strips, and lancets to prick your finger. (All are available without a prescription at most big-box stores and pharmacies for around $25. Many doctors' offices also make them available without charge—just ask.) It will take a few minutes to get acquainted with your device by following the instructions provided with the device. Alternatively, one of the continuous glucose monitors (CGMs) that provide real-time blood sugars can accomplish the same without need for finger pricks. Devices are also now obtainable on your own without your doctor's participation.

Start by obtaining a reading immediately prior to a meal. Start your meal, then obtain another measure thirty to sixty minutes after the start, a so-called postprandial measure. We aim for *no change*. For example, if the initial measure is 100 mg/dl, we want the second during-meal measure to be no higher than 100 mg/dl—no change (accepting that the readings are accurate to +/– 10 mg/dl. No change would therefore fall in the range of 90 to 110 mg/dl.). If your during-meal reading is, say, 136 mg/dl, look at your meal and identify the carbohydrate culprit. The next time you eat a similar meal, cut back on portion size or eliminate the culprit food altogether. By doing so repeatedly, you will accelerate loss of abdominal fat and weight loss, and reduce both fasting and postprandial blood sugars. Over time, by adhering to this no-change rule, premeal or fasting blood sugar levels will usually also drop into the ideal range of 60 to 90 mg/dl.

Ignore critics who say, "That's not how to measure blood sugars. You're supposed to check your sugar two hours after a meal." This is the rule people are advised to follow to determine whether blood sugars return to baseline levels while on insulin and other blood glucose–reducing medications—that, of course, is *not* our concern. Recall that we also ignore advice from doctors who declare, "Any blood glucose of ≤200 mg/dl is fine," as this is simply untrue. A blood glucose of, say, 160 mg/dl is more than enough to trigger insulin and expansion of abdominal fat, as well as collagen glycation and formation of small LDL particles that cause heart disease. By keeping all blood sugars ≤100 mg/dl, you avoid all these phenomena.

There is no need to conduct this little exercise indefinitely. You will likely find that, after testing over a couple of weeks, you will quickly recognize problem foods and what foods are safe.

Drink filtered water—It's a two-edged sword: Most cities filter water to remove unwanted contaminants, but water filtration is also extremely efficient at removing minerals we need for health, especially magnesium, iodine, potassium, and calcium. But drinking filtered water, or water obtained from other safe sources, is a modern necessity if we are to be protected from contaminating microbes, pesticides, herbicides, heavy metals such as lead and cadmium, and other common water contaminants. Think: Flint, Michigan, with lead contamination, or Milwaukee, Wisconsin, with a *Cryptosporidium* outbreak. Given the size and complexity of our society, drinking unfiltered water is downright dangerous.

Unfortunately, there is an added layer of challenge with drinking water. City water treatment facilities add chlorine or chloramine to kill microbial contaminants, and fluoride to prevent tooth decay, compounds with antimicrobial properties upon consumption. Preliminary evidence suggests that these chemicals disrupt the gastrointestinal mucus barrier that, in turn, can change the composition of bacteria in the microbiome. In other words, even though your city filters your water, it unwittingly adds to your health challenges because—despite good intentions—such treatments introduce factors that change the microbiome.[25] While further research is required to understand the full microbiome and health implications of these practices, it appears likely that they add further to your health, microbiome, and body contour woes.

I therefore urge everyone to add a water filtration system in their home. It could be an inexpensive filtered pitcher you keep on your kitchen counter that uses charcoal to filter out contaminants, or the water dispenser on your refrigerator. It could be a reverse osmosis and/or charcoal filtration system that filters water coming out of your kitchen tap, or a basement system that filters all household water, including the water you use to shower or bathe. As with the modern diet that has become a barrier to your health and body-reshaping efforts, so it has gone with water also. The maneuver of filtering your water can serve as a simple solution.

Follow these guidelines and you will be able to mimic, as best as possible in our electronic world, the diet programmed into your forty-six chromosomes. You will find yourself shopping almost exclusively in the meat and produce departments, rarely needing to venture into the inner aisles stacked with processed foods and soft drinks. Sure, you might have to venture into those aisles for laundry detergent or paper towels, but there is almost nothing in those aisles safe to eat. Among the few exceptions: salsas, extra-virgin olive oil, nuts, seeds, spices. But recognize that you are venturing into enemy territory, fraught with unhealthy land mines ready to destroy your health and create abnormal bulges and protuberances. To help you navigate this lifestyle, see the summary I've assembled in Appendix A.

LOST NUTRIENTS

This chapter is surely enough to keep you busy and engaged for the first week. Let's discuss in Chapter 8 how and why we supplement nutrients lacking or absent in modern life that also play outsize roles in determining shape and body composition. During Week 2 of the program, you will therefore add several nutrients to the benefits of the diet you have adopted, magnifying effects on shrinking abdominal visceral fat, reducing insulin resistance and inflammation, helping rebuild lost muscle, and further improving body contours.

8

WEEK 2:
SUN, WATER, AND SEA:
LOST NATURAL FACTORS
THAT SHAPE YOUR BODY

IN WEEK 2, LET'S CONSIDER THE NUTRIENTS LACKING FROM your comfortable modern life that would have been obtained had you hunted, foraged, or dug for food and water that, when restored, add to your body-shaping efforts.

To understand what I mean, let's return to our make-believe world of 50,000 BC. You have just awoken from sleep, the fire from the evening before is now just embers. You grab a spear and perhaps your atlatl, an ancient device that propels the spear with great force and velocity. On your way to hunting grounds you previously identified as abundantly inhabited with wildlife, you stop to drink deeply from a stream where water runs freely over rocks and minerals. You spy some crawfish and mussels that you gather and consume raw. Clad only in a loincloth and loosely fitting fur over your torso, as well as skins covering your feet, you feel the sun's rays on your exposed abdomen, head, legs, and arms. You occasionally stop to consume some plant matter or fruit that you stumble across. Although tough and fibrous, it helps beat back the hunger as you walk and run several miles during the hunt.

You arrive at the foot of a mountain where you have seen wild goats congregate in the past. You spot a small herd, including one member that is clearly injured and limping—an easy target. You and your fellow hunters spread out to cut off any chance of escape. You stealthily approach the animals, but the herd detects your presence and scatters. Two of your clan members lie in waiting, one launching the spear on his atlatl that pierces the side of the weakened goat, causing it to run for several minutes, then collapse. You approach, finishing off the animal by cutting its throat with your stone knife. You and your fellow hunters slice open its abdomen and consume some of the liver, raw and bloody. Satiated, you drag the carcass along the grass several miles back to camp, where the rest of your clan cheer, getting the fire ready to cook the meat and organs.

Sun, water, wild fruits and plants, crustaceans and shellfish, organ meats—this is the lifestyle to which you and your ancestors have adapted, providing all the nutrients you require for a long and healthy life, barring injury and infections carried, for instance, by mosquitoes or flies. You enjoy a muscled, flat abdomen, strong sinewy arms and legs. There is no abdominal protuberance, no ectopic fat degrading hips and knees, but muscle that makes it possible to run, climb, hunt, or just dig in the dirt for roots and tubers. Your skin has been tanned by daily exposure to sun over much of your body surface area that activates vitamin D. You obtained such minerals as magnesium, calcium, sodium, iron, and copper by drinking from freely running water and consuming wild plants. You have no qualms about sharing a slice of brain from the animal you killed, rich in omega-3 fatty acids and hyaluronic acid, or the tongue and heart rich in collagen. You are careful to share a small piece of thyroid with all clan members, as you know those who do not partake will experience a disfiguring goiter, later succumbing to a body grotesquely disfigured from edema and fat and, eventually, death (myxedema from lack of iodine). No one here adheres to dietary guidelines, no one is counting calories, no one is concerned about fat or cholesterol intake. There are no ads to persuade you that some manufactured product is somehow preferable to your habitual diet, nor are you tempted by flashy packaging or discount coupons.

Everything you need to survive comes to you from your lifestyle with freely accessible air and water, hunting and scavenging for sustenance, living the way that has been programmed over many generations into the genetic code of *Homo sapiens*.

It was not that long ago that our great-grandparents, living many tens of thousands of years later than our 50,000 BC world, were clothed in naturally sourced materials, many of which they sewed or wove themselves. Their foods were purchased at the butcher who sold only freshly slaughtered meats and organs, as well as meats he fermented in his cellar or back room. While people of that age relied on their own gardens for much of their vegetables, fruit trees and vines for fruit, the nearby river for shellfish, their diet habits had evolved compared to that of their ancestors of 50,000 BC. But the foods they chose did not yet include preservatives, emulsifying agents, loads of sugar, or synthetic sweeteners. There was no such thing as "fast food," no drive-thru windows, no ready-made deli dishes, no delivering restaurant food in a clamshell, no food plates or pyramids to tell them how to manage eating habits. In fact, it was likely that they churned their own butter, butchered their own pigs, and fermented vegetables in their basement.

I detail all this to emphasize just how perverse our modern notion of diet has become. It took a half century of dietary blundering, a.k.a. "dietary guidelines" and the unrestrained proliferation of ultraprocessed foods, to teach us how far we have veered off course from a diet that is natural and provides nutrients whose needs are programmed into our genetic code.

I fear that, for many of us, there is no going back. Your great-grandmother may have sucked the marrow out of bones or deftly chopped the heads off chickens before removing feathers and retrieving liver, gizzard, and feet. But we have become so accustomed to modern conveniences that the thought of roasting tongue or frying up some skin is repulsive to most of us. But our modern revulsion means that we are deprived of nutrients crucial to body shape and composition as well as health.

It's no news that modern people like their nutritional supplements. But most of the supplements that people take do not follow any specific rhyme or reason as part of a more comprehensive and logical approach to address intrinsic human need. Let's instead restore factors that should have come from a natural diet of hunting and gathering, of drinking from rivers and streams, of living outdoors in a tropical or semitropical climate, a lifestyle that shaped human adaptation. In other words, we are not introducing factors that are foreign to the human experience; we are *restoring* factors that should have been part of your life all along. We therefore resist the idea of "treating" abnormal phenomena, such as high blood sugar, high blood pressure, or fatty liver. Instead, we are going to address factors that allow such phenomena to appear in the first place.

I shall therefore address:

- Vitamin D—lacking because of living our lives indoors, wearing clothing that covers much skin surface area, and other factors. You may already know that restoration of vitamin D is important for such issues as bone health or protection from winter "blues." But you may not know that it is also an important ingredient in your effort to restructure the shape of your body.
- Minerals and micronutrients lacking in modern life— Magnesium and iodine are among the most important.
- Nutrients lacking due to our aversion to consumption of organ meats—We've already considered collagen and hyaluronic acid, so let's focus on omega-3 fatty acids.

As unconnected as this collection of nutrients seems, when addressed as a whole, they create a combination that reverses or minimizes body-shaping phenomena, such as insulin resistance and inflammation. Add the body-composition effects experienced by restoring specific bacterial species, microbes lost from the majority of gastrointestinal tracts of modern humans, and you have the key to shrinking abdominal visceral fat and thereby waist circumference, followed by reduced subcutaneous fat in buttocks, thighs, arms, and elsewhere, while increasing lean muscle mass, shifting your bulges to places you'd prefer to have them. Combine all the factors discussed and a powerful synergy develops.

Let's begin with this absolutely essential factor to human existence: exposure to sunlight.

SUNSHINE: ENERGY OF LIFE

A life outdoors in a tropical or semitropical climate, scantily clad with plenty of exposed skin surface area, allows the activation of vitamin D in the skin upon sun exposure. Vitamin D—crucial for so many body systems, from enhancing the immune response to allowing your body to respond to insulin, to maintaining bone and muscle—is meant to be largely obtained by living your life bathed in the natural ultraviolet wavelengths of sunlight. Dietary sources of vitamin D are meager; a small quantity can be obtained from consumption of animal organs, some fish, birds' eggs, and from the plant form of vitamin D_2 (though not as effective as the animal source, D_3) from consumption of mushrooms. Without sun there would be no life. Vitamin D is therefore one of the key ways that the energy of the sun is transmitted into your body, allowing your complex multicellular physiology to operate and thrive in a sun-soaked environment. Without a source of vitamin D, you increase your risk of tooth decay, cancer, bone thinning, heart disease, complications of pregnancy and delivery, distortions of body shape—in short, a life cut short or filled with major health struggles and diminished hopes for survival.[1]

Ah, but you live in a northern climate. Or you work indoors, perhaps remotely, emerging from your apartment or home to shop in an air-conditioned or heated supermarket, getting there in an air-conditioned or heated motor vehicle. Like most law-abiding citizens, you wear clothes covering much of your skin surface area whenever you are outdoors. You may be among the 35 percent of Americans with fatty liver or the 108 million Americans who are obese, situations that cause more severe degrees of vitamin D deficiency and require greater quantities of the nutrient to achieve healthy blood levels.[2] And you are aging, gradually losing the ability to activate vitamin D in the skin, obtaining little even with a dark tan after age forty. Modern people are therefore miserably vitamin D deficient. Restoration of vitamin D can provide relief from disparate health phenomena while also making a contribution to helping you gain control over distorted body contours. Vitamin D by itself makes a major contribution to overall health, but in the context of shape and body composition, it is part of a synergistic mix of factors we are going to restore.

VITAMIN D: SEEING THE LIGHT

My personal experience with vitamin D was eye-opening, a lesson I learned during my many years of being immersed in a busy cardiology medical practice.

Practicing cardiology can be an around-the-clock affair. It wasn't uncommon to wake up at two or three a.m. for an emergency, or at five a.m. for an early-morning procedure. I have memories of many nights of waking up in the dark, feeling an oppressive weight on my shoulders, sometimes standing in the shower as the water washed over me, wondering why I chose to subject myself to such a torturous schedule.

But then I learned of the effects of vitamin D. I had been thinking and writing about vitamin D. An article I wrote about vitamin D caught the attention of Dr. John Cannell, a psychiatrist from California who devoted his efforts to broadcasting the idea that vitamin D deficiency was a health problem of epidemic proportions and how restoring it was incredibly powerful and easy. Dr. Cannell made a career out of educating physicians and the public on the need for vitamin D. I therefore put myself on 10,000 units per day.

The effects for me were nothing short of miraculous. Showering at five a.m., dark as night outside, I felt elated and freed, none of the dark feelings and oppression I had suffered in previous years. I felt more alive, more upbeat, more alert. At the time, I was living in Wisconsin, where it can be winter nearly six months a year, a latitude that made getting plentiful intense sunlight every day impossible. I was therefore deeply grateful to learn that I could enjoy this way of mimicking many of the effects of sunlight.

As I incorporated advice to increase vitamin D intake in my patients, I again witnessed significant and sometimes extraordinary effects. Among the many wonderful experiences related to me by my patients was one man, being seen for coronary disease, whose father-in-law lived in his home. His father-in-law had dementia, his days occupied by simply sitting in front of the TV from morning until bedtime. My patient's wife began supplementing vitamin D to her father. My patient said that, one morning a short time later, he saw his father-in-law whiz past a window, on a riding lawn mower, cutting the grass. He described how, while still showing signs of dementia, his father-in-law had, to a surprising degree, "reawakened" from the advanced dementia he'd been experiencing. It's not a cure for such conditions, of course, but what else can provide such wonderful effects, so safely, so inexpensively, simply by addressing a natural need?

Given its enormous importance for health, and the significant advantages in achieving a healthy blood level of vitamin D—a blood level of 25-OH vitamin D, the primary indicator of the vitamin's status—you would expect practicing physicians to be experts in vitamin D. But that's not how the world works. You likely know that if something does not yield substantial payoffs to a physician or health-care system, it receives little attention. Statin cholesterol drugs that achieve almost nothing in reducing cardiovascular risk but generate billions of dollars per year for the pharmaceutical industry? They receive plenty of attention. Bariatric surgical procedures that, with better information, are largely unnecessary and often harmful but yield substantial professional and procedural fees? Plenty of popular press. But a nutrient that, when replaced, yields huge health benefits but costs almost nothing and does not generate any payoffs to doctors or hospitals? Good luck trying to get informed answers from your doctor.

So, what can vitamin D do for all the bulges and protuberances we have? Plenty. But just as a day in the sun will not reverse all distorted body contours, it is just one piece of the puzzle—a critical piece that, when combined with correction of dietary deficiencies and missing microbes, has potential to not just make you happier and less inflamed but also help you reduce abdominal fat and regain youthful muscle. Vitamin D helps achieve these desired body-reshaping benefits because it reduces insulin resistance that regulates abdominal fat while also reducing age-related loss of muscle.[3] Just as I call oxytocin "the hormone of shape and body composition" because of its spectacular effects on fat and muscle, so we could call vitamin D "the nutrient of body composition." Although not as powerful as oxytocin, vitamin D's power comes when we correct deficiencies of other factors with effects amplified by this vitamin.

SEEING RED

Upon exposure to sunlight, it is the shorter wavelength ultra-violet (UV) light that activates vitamin D in the skin. It is also UV light that causes tanning and sunburns. The short wave-length of UV light means that it is incapable of penetrating any further than less than one millimeter of the skin.

Infrared (IR) light is at the opposite end of the spectrum, with much longer wavelengths more powerful in penetrating the skin. It has been shown to penetrate deep into the body, passing through clothing and even completely through the body. Sunlight provides plenty of light from the IR end of the spectrum. Recent research has demonstrated that IR light that penetrates into the body has the unique ability to increase the number and activity of mitochondria, the energy-producing organelles within your body's cells, especially in the brain, retina, and muscle. Dr. Glen Jeffery of University

College, London, conducted a unique study in which human participants underwent a glucose tolerance test after IR exposure. Participants were given a large quantity of sugar, then blood glucose was tracked over 120 minutes. Participants wore blindfolds and received either IR light or no light to their upper backs. Surprisingly, participants receiving IR light showed 27 percent lower glucose levels (integrated over two hours), while also increasing the release of carbon dioxide on their breath, indicating accelerated metabolism of sugars.[4]

Conversely, other studies have shown that exposure to light wavelengths (450 nm) produced by popular light-emitting diode (LED) lightbulbs, light more toward the opposite or blue end of the light spectrum, achieves the opposite: increased insulin resistance.[5] Recall that insulin resistance is the phenomenon that adds to expansion of abdominal visceral fat, loss of muscle, myosteatosis, and other forms of ectopic fat.

Therefore, consider:

- Living an indoor lifestyle with little to no exposure to IR wavelengths likely adds to insulin resistance and all its consequences.
- Exposure to LED blue wavelength light adds further to insulin resistance, especially with exposure later in the day.

In short, exposure to sunlight improves factors influencing location of fat and muscle, while exposure to indoor LED lighting does the opposite.

It is yet another example of how living our lives like our ancestors, who enjoyed plentiful exposure to sunlight and, of course, no LED lighting in their huts or caves, will likely add to our capacity to regulate shape and body composition.

So, yes, vitamin D is important and yields numerous health benefits. Combining vitamin D with exposure to sunlight and, when such exposure is not possible due to weather, climate, latitude, or schedule, exposure to IR light (e.g., 670 nm wavelength) may add further to your ability to control shape and body composition. (See Appendix D for recommended devices.) And if your life is like mine, in which I

spend many hours every day looking at a computer screen
with most lightbulbs in the house of the LED variety (both
sources of blue wavelength), in addition to sunlight and/or IR
light, consider switching back to old-fashioned incandescent
bulbs at your desk that provide additional IR spectrum light
and wearing blue-blocking glasses to reduce exposure to the
blue wavelength that can damage eye structures.

We therefore supplement vitamin D (and perhaps add some sun
exposure while avoiding sunburn) to achieve an ideal blood level, such
as that experienced by people who live their lives outdoors. Just as
obtaining drinking water from a river or stream poses health haz-
ards, and eating fish every day likewise introduces heavy metal exposure risks, so does obtaining excessive sunlight to activate vitamin D,
given the depletion of the ozone layer of the upper atmosphere that
has increased the intensity of ultraviolet radiation responsible for acti-
vating vitamin D in the skin but also increasing risk for skin cancer.
Once again, we therefore resort to a safe oral work-around in the form
of vitamin D supplementation, with daily exposure to some sunlight,
never allowing sunburn and minimizing your exposure to LED wavelengths of light.

I advocate restoring vitamin D only in oil-based gelcap form for
assured absorption, not powder in capsule or tablet forms that are
erratically absorbed, sometimes not absorbed at all. And you should
only supplement the human form, cholecalciferol (D_3), and never the
plant form, ergocalciferol (D_2), as the D_2 does not raise blood levels
nor bind to vitamin D receptors in various organs as well as D_3.[6] I also
discourage "bolus" dosing, such as 50,000 units per week or 100,000
units per month, as the evidence suggests that most of the benefits of
this nutrient are reduced or lost completely when taken this way (likely
by being routed through a different metabolic pathway).[7] The most

common challenge with vitamin D is knowing what dose to take—most people are afraid to take the dose necessary to obtain full benefit.

WHAT IS AN IDEAL VITAMIN D BLOOD LEVEL?

When I asked patients in my cardiology practice to supplement vitamin D, I first obtained a baseline level prior to supplementation. A starting value of 25-OH vitamin D of 15 ng/ml was typical. The laboratory report at the time stated that the reference range (the range that the laboratory recommended) was 10 to 20 ng/ml. Yet the emerging experience suggested that levels more toward 60 ng/ml were associated with a long list of health benefits. Why the difference?

To illustrate, let's pretend that you ask me, "What's the average weight of a woman in my part of the country?" So I propose that you and I go to the local mall. We politely stop every woman who walks by and ask to anonymously measure her body weight with a scale we've brought. After weighing a thousand women, we tally up our numbers. We find that the average weight for adult women in our area is 176 pounds with variation (standard deviation) of +/−25 pounds (which is typical for many areas of the country). Would you interpret this as "normal" or ideal? Probably not. It is a *population average*. But this is how laboratories generate many of their "reference ranges." In the case of vitamin D, many labs obtained their reference range values by testing a population that lacks sun exposure and does not supplement vitamin D and is thereby guaranteed to be deficient—yet that is the basis for what doctors regard as "normal." They fail to ask, "What is optimal?"

So let's ask that question ourselves. By examining the evidence, we can surmise that:

- Epidemiologically, there is a sharp drop-off in cancer incidence in people with 25-OH vitamin D blood levels above 50 ng/ml.[8]

- If you were an eighteen-year-old lifeguard in Honolulu—that is, young and thereby retaining the ability to activate vitamin D in the skin and exposed to tropical sun over a large skin surface area—it would not be unexpected to have a 25-OH vitamin D blood level in the 80s ng/ml or even 90 ng/ml, suggesting that this is a physiologically achievable, appropriate, and safe level.[9]
- When vitamin D levels are low, there is increased release of parathyroid hormone (PTH) from the parathyroid glands that causes you to extract calcium from your bones that leads over time to bone thinning (osteopenia, osteoporosis). What level of 25-OH vitamin D is required to maximally suppress PTH, to thereby protect your bones? Fifty ng/ml or greater.[10]

Given this evidence, I have been advocating that we achieve a 25-OH vitamin D level of 60 to 70 ng/ml. After having accomplished this in thousands of patients, I have never witnessed a single case of toxicity, yet did witness many wonderful health benefits by achieving levels significantly higher than the laboratory "reference range."

TROUBLED WATERS

Before modern waterways became contaminated with farm runoff, sewage, and industrial waste, water was like air, something we had easy access to, a necessity that was reliable and clean. Freely running fresh water, flowing over rocks, minerals, sand, and soil, was therefore rich in nutrients.

Drink from a stream or river today, however, and you are likely to have diarrhea or something worse. In our modern world, we must therefore filter drinking water. Your city filters the water before it comes out of your tap while also adding such chemicals as chlorine or chloramine to kill contaminating fecal microbes. Or perhaps you filter it in your home with a basement or kitchen water filter, a countertop filtration device, or you rely on bottled water. Nearly all these forms of water retain little to no magnesium or other minerals, as water filtration is exceptionally efficient at removing minerals to convert "hard" water to "soft" and to minimize exposure to pathogens and toxins. It also means that you no longer obtain any significant quantities of minerals through the simple act of drinking water. We also know that magnesium content of produce such as cabbage, lettuce, tomatoes, and spinach is 80–90 percent less than it was a century ago.[11] The cabbage you serve today is a shadow, nutritionally speaking, of cabbage soup or fermented sauerkraut of a century ago.

Of all the minerals lacking because you filter drinking water, the most important is magnesium. Low tissue and blood levels of magnesium can be dangerous, even life-threatening. In my cardiology days, people who developed unstable and potentially fatal heart rhythms (e.g., torsades de pointes, or ventricular tachycardia) would be given intravenous magnesium with miraculous results literally within moments. Pregnant women experiencing eclampsia or preeclampsia with high blood pressure and risk of seizure, situations that put the lives of both mother and baby at risk, are treated with intravenous magnesium. Go to the emergency room with an incapacitating migraine headache, and an intravenous magnesium infusion is among the first treatments offered. In other words, the need for magnesium to control numerous physiologic processes is unquestioned, able to remedy crippling or even potentially fatal processes. These situations are brought about, at least in part, by magnesium deficiency.[12,13]

Because we must filter our drinking water and rarely eat wild plants rich in minerals and, even worse, consume wheat and grains that contain phytates that bind magnesium in the gut, causing us to pass minerals into the toilet, magnesium deficiency is rampant and severe. But it should not take a fatal heart rhythm or a dangerous pregnancy situation to tell you that you have a deficiency of this important mineral. Just by living your everyday life, drinking filtered water, eating food purchased in a supermarket, and including "healthy whole grains" in your diet, you can be certain that you lack magnesium. But don't fall into the trap of believing that because your blood test for magnesium, a "serum magnesium," was in the reference range that your magnesium status must therefore be fine.[11] Because magnesium is so crucial to keep your heart beating normally and many other critical functions, your body protects this important serum level. Because the serum level is "protected" to keep you from these dangerous events, your body will extract huge quantities of magnesium from such places as bones, the primary repository for magnesium, to protect your serum level. You won't know that you are magnesium deficient by measuring serum levels until it's too late and you end up on the receiving end of a defibrillator. You therefore want a *tissue* level, not a serum level. But no one wants to undergo a biopsy of an organ to obtain a tissue level, so we go with second-best: a red blood cell (RBC) magnesium.[14] This is the measurement you are most interested in. And you want this value to be toward the upper range of the reference range. If your laboratory quotes a reference range of, say, 4.8 to 6.2 mg/dl, you want a level of 6.0 mg/dl or higher (though probably no higher than 6.8 mg/dl—the optimal upper limit has not yet been established).[15] But note that, even with supplementation of 450 to 500 mg of magnesium per day, it can take one or two *years* to see your RBC magnesium level rise. But with the rise in magnesium, you are likely to experience reduced blood pressure, reduced heart rhythm issues, freedom from muscle cramps, reduced blood sugar, and improved bone health.

Magnesium carries implications for your shape and body composition ambitions, since it helps reduce insulin resistance.[16,17] Magnesium also makes a contribution to the loss of abdominal fat and increasing muscle.[18] Once again, the real benefits of magnesium show, when experienced in the context of all the other strategies discussed here, a powerful synergistic combination.

ROUGH SEAS

Sea water contains plenty of the trace mineral iodine, as do animals or plants living in the sea: fish, shellfish, kelp, and other ocean fauna, as well as plants and animals that grow or live along coastal shores, where iodine leaches into the soil. Creatures from the sea are also rich in omega-3 fatty acids, fats crucial for human health, especially since most modern people have abandoned consumption of organ meats from land animals. Therefore, let's now consider these two ocean-sourced nutrients important for serving your body-shape ambitions.

Over many generations, many human populations have migrated to mountainous or inland parts of every continent, far away from iodine sources. Some iodine could be obtained by consumption of the thyroid glands of animals, but the farther from the ocean a population of humans migrated, the more likely deficiency of this trace mineral became. Iodine deficiency has therefore been one of the most widespread public health problems that has plagued our species for much of human history. Inland populations, such as those in the American Midwest, or mountainous villages in Europe, or inland parts of Africa, therefore suffered epidemics of disfiguring goiters, enlarged thyroid glands on the front of the neck reflecting the thyroid gland's effort to better extract iodine from the bloodstream. Over time, this growth could suffocate by crushing the trachea (windpipe). More commonly, lack of iodine meant that the thyroid was unable to produce sufficient quantities of thyroid hormone. The sufferer gained fat weight due to slowed metabolism, retained huge quantities of water resulting in grotesque degrees of edema, and finally died of either heart failure or coma. If you could ask your great-grandmother if she remembers the days of goiters, she would likely respond, "Oh, yes, it was awful. My fourth-grade teacher had a goiter so large that she had to carry it in her arms until she died. Three of my classmates in high school had to drop out because they gained so much weight and could no longer walk, and then died." In mountainous parts of Europe, there were entire villages of dwarflike residents with impaired intelligence and goiters, whom people labeled "cretins," all due to lack of iodine.[19]

This all began to change when, in 1924, proof emerged demonstrating that a deficiency of the micronutrient iodine was to blame. Programs were introduced to provide iodine to schoolchildren, and a public health campaign was launched in which salt manufacturers were encouraged to add iodine to salt, the public then encouraged to consume plenty of salt. Posters were put up in public places: "Use more iodized salt. Keep your family goiter-free." Another half century passed and, coupled with widespread advice to reduce fat and cholesterol and increase consumption of grain products, greater struggles with hypertension and other health problems increased, a situation that the Food and Drug Administration (FDA) interpreted as evidence of salt overuse. They therefore reversed their advice of fifty years earlier and urged Americans to slash salt intake. The American Heart Association (AHA) and other dietary agencies urged Americans to reduce sodium intake to levels as low as 1,500 milligrams per day (1 teaspoon salt = 2,300 mg sodium), a level that made food virtually unpalatable and, of course, limited iodine.[19,20]

Despite the huge public health success of the "use more iodized salt" campaign, the more recent advice has caused—not surprisingly—a return of iodine deficiency and even goiters.[21] Although not as bad as it was pre-1924, likely due to the globalization of the food supply—you get tomatoes from California, avocados from Mexico, bananas from Brazil, and so on—the blame placed on iodized salt has caused a resurgence of thyroid dysfunction that further contributes to distortions of weight and body composition.

WRONGLY ACCUSED

The shift away from fats and toward increased carbohydrate intake that began in the 1970s and increased in earnest in the 1980s brought with it an explosion in insulin resistance—poor responsiveness of muscle, brain, liver, and other organs to insulin, such that 70 percent of the US population today is insulin resistant, teenagers and children included (with varied estimates due to varying definitions).[22] Ironically, the repeated cycles of high blood glucose and high blood insulin that result from an increase in dietary carbohydrates and sugars cause the cells of the body to block entry of glucose. In this situation, the pancreas receives a signal that blood glucose is becoming unavailable to the body's organs and that it should produce more insulin. Insulin blood levels therefore increase ten-, fifty-, even a hundredfold, a situation that causes not only expansion of fat stores and loss of muscle but also retention of sodium by the kidneys, thus the apparent problem with sodium.[23] And yet a further irony: Restricting sodium also makes insulin resistance worse, thereby worsening sodium retention by the kidneys. In other words, the purported "solution" to a problem, consistent with the continued pattern of blundering in dietary guidelines, inadvertently worsened the problem.[24]

I hope that you now appreciate that blame was misplaced. Salt and sodium were innocent bystanders in a process resulting from an unnatural distortion of diet caused by flawed advice, then worsened by the proliferation of ultraprocessed foods, two factors that conspired to cause sodium retention. Rather than provide advice to consume foods in their natural form, extreme advice emerged, such as the AHA's fatally restrictive advice. More recent analyses of the effects of this and similar levels of sodium restriction suggest that curtailing sodium intake to extremes like this not only makes life miserable but also increases mortality and shortens life span.[25,26] While some of the advice emerging from this experience was useful, such as to reduce consumption of fast food, ultraprocessed food, and soft drinks, it also generated plenty of useless advice in managing salt intake. Anyone engaging in such extremes of sodium restriction will readily tell you that foods minus salt take away all the pleasures of taste. Soups are bland, meats unappealing. Vegetables lose their flavor that might have been salvaged by adding butter but—nope, stay away from butter too, the AHA says.

Time and time again, conventional sources of dietary information got it wrong, tragically wrong.

A return to iodine can involve iodized salt, though you may prefer to use either kelp (dried seaweed) tablets or potassium iodide drops, both available and inexpensive. While iodized salt can serve as a source and was indeed successful in eradicating goiters for many decades as a public health maneuver, be aware that, once a salt canister is opened, iodine volatilizes; that is, it evaporates into the air as iodine gas, and the container no longer has any iodine in it four weeks after opening.[27] The Recommended Daily Allowance for iodine is 150 mcg per day for an adult, a recommendation based on the amount of iodine needed to not have a goiter. Instead, I advise a higher intake, in the range of 300 to 450 mcg/day, which I believe is more in line with the optimal range for production of thyroid hormones and protection from ubiquitous industrial compounds, such as perfluorooctanoic acid from Teflon or triclosan in hand sanitizers.[28,29]

Another factor that has nearly disappeared from the human diet sourced from the sea is omega-3 fatty acids, eicosopentaenoic acid (EPA) and docosahexaenoic acid (DHA). As mentioned earlier, consumption of the brains of animals yields abundant quantities of omega-3s, especially DHA (explaining why, for instance, omega-3 intake is crucial in preventing cognitive impairment and Alzheimer's and other forms of dementia[30]). But, of course, few modern people are willing to incorporate brain matter into their daily routine. Other factors such as limited availability and prion diseases complicate the situation. So, folding some chopped sheep or cow brain into your scrambled eggs, a common practice a century ago, is no longer a good idea. Likewise, alternative sources of omega-3s, seafood and shellfish, are now contaminated with heavy metals, specifically mercury and cadmium, making consumption of more than occasional servings hazardous. These metals are poorly cleared by the body and thereby accumulate over time, building up risk for health conditions that include dementia, kidney disease, and various cancers.[31]

We are left with supplementing with fish oil. The process of extracting and purifying oils from fish yields oils that have negligible quantities of contaminants.[32] In general, the best policy is to obtain nutrients from their original source, food intact. But most of us have little or no control over issues like widespread industrialization and contamination of the food supply, so we resort to purified EPA and

DHA from fish oil for omega-3 fatty acids necessary for numerous health benefits, as well as contributing to our shape and body composition efforts. Among the effects of omega-3 fatty acids that help reduce abdominal fat and waist size, help maintain or build muscle, and thereby restore or maintain youthful body composition are:

- Reduction in breakdown products from unhealthy gut microbes—The entry of bacterial breakdown products into the bloodstream, an important and underappreciated process labeled "endotoxemia" (that I will discuss at greater length in Chapter 9), is a major driver of insulin resistance and inflammation that provokes expansion of abdominal visceral fat and impairs muscle. Omega-3s make a contribution to reducing this phenomenon.[33]

- The several hours after a meal, the so-called postprandial period, is characterized by the entry of various fat-carrying proteins (lipoproteins) into the bloodstream. These lipoproteins, especially those derived from carbohydrate and sugar consumption, add further to insulin resistance and inflammation that drive abdominal fat accumulation. Omega-3 fatty acids reduce lipoproteins significantly.[34]

- The modern diet has included a shift away from omega-3 fatty acid sources and become overloaded with omega-6 fatty acids, due to overconsumption of processed oils such as corn, mixed "vegetable," sunflower, cottonseed, and safflower oils. The combination of lack of omega-3s coupled with overconsumption of omega-6s has worsened insulin resistance and inflammation, adding to both accumulation of abdominal fat and erosion of muscle.[35] (But don't make the mistake of avoiding omega-6 fats altogether as they are also essential, just necessary at much lower intakes.)

In short, omega-3 fatty acids sourced from fish oil—not the plant-sourced omega-3 (linolenic acid) from such foods as flaxseeds and chia seeds, which while beneficial do not mimic the effects of EPA and

DHA,[36] nor does krill oil, often misleadingly marketed as a superior supplement to fish oil but contains only minor amounts of omega-3s—are the fatty acids that you need with wide health benefits that, in the context of all the other strategies I discuss here, add to youth-restoring, body-contouring effects. For the purposes of maximizing the contribution of omega-3 fatty acids to reshaping body contours, the dose we aim for is a minimum of 3,000 mg per day of the combination of EPA and DHA—not the intake of fish oil, but of the EPA and DHA contained. If, for example, you buy a product in which one capsule provides 360 mg of EPA and 240 mg of DHA, each capsule therefore provides 360 mg + 240 mg = 600 mg. Five capsules per day (that can be divided) or more is the effective dose, ideally divided into two doses (e.g., with breakfast and an afternoon meal).

PARADISE REVISITED

We are embarking on a journey to restore human life to something closer to the way it was supposed to be. No, we cannot freely drink water from rivers or streams. Most of us cannot enjoy prolonged exposure to tropical or subtropical sun with plenty of surface area exposed, or we are beyond the age that yields full benefit. And it is impossible to know the iodine content of most foods, nor do many of us want to risk eating foods from the ocean in unlimited quantities due to industrial contamination, and most modern people do not relish the idea of returning to cracking open an animal's skull to harvest the brain, or sucking on bones to access the marrow, or frying up a slice of liver.

We endeavor to restore nutrients that mimic these lost factors, all of which play important roles in reestablishing control over your body size and contours, bringing back the muscular, nonprotuberant shape that humans previously enjoyed.

In the third week of this program, let's explore one of the most fascinating areas to emerge from the evolving science of health: the role of the gastrointestinal microbiome in shaping your body contours.

9

WEEK 3:
CELEBRATE THE BODY-SHAPING POWER OF THE GUT-MUSCLE AXIS

You MAKE THOUSANDS OF DECISIONS EVERY DAY: WHAT TO wear, who to talk to, what to say, what to eat, what to buy, among many others. It leads you to believe that, in a democratic society filled with spectacular freedoms, you are the ultimate decision maker. Psychologists tell us that self-determination is the key to happiness; politicians running for office give us wide choices in policy; our consumerist society provides incredible variety in buying power.

Ah, but you have been given a half-truth. Yes, you can indeed make your own decisions, but they are influenced to an astounding degree by the trillions of microscopic creatures you harbor in your body. Anonymous, without names, and dismissed with derogatory terms such as *crap* and *sh—*, pooh-poohed by most doctors as nothing more than a nuisance that causes diarrhea after a course of antibiotics, the several pounds of microbes you harbor in the 30 feet of your GI tract and other organs influence every aspect of your life. They influence mood and the success or failure of relationships; they play a role in determining whether you are able to bear children, whether your children will be delivered prematurely or at full term, whether you are a law-abiding taxpaying citizen or someone driven by hate who chooses to gun down unarmed people in a crowd.[1] I cannot overstate the power that the communities of microbes in your body's microbiome play in your life and the lives of those around you.

You now know that modern life has negatively impacted the composition of microbes housed in your body. As I've discussed, numerous factors have led to a dramatic shift in the species that live in the modern human GI tract. Compared to the few remaining hunter-gatherer populations unexposed to such factors, the microbial composition of our colons is unrecognizably different: They have microbial species we don't have; we possess species they do not, and they have a wider variety of microbes, a virtual lush tropical jungle of diverse species compared to our dry, desiccated desert. The microbial populations we harbor in our colons are different from those carried by people living the lifestyle that preceded our industrialized lives. This alone carries implications for such conditions as constipation, hemorrhoids, ulcerative colitis, prostate disease, and colon cancer.[2]

In this third week of our effort to redistribute your body contours, let's explore the critical and powerful role of the GI microbiome. It is the last collection of strategies we consider, admittedly a bit more complicated than the previous two weeks. Invest a little time and effort, however, and you will be rewarded with a degree of control over health, shape, and body composition that you may not have thought was possible.

LOCATION, LOCATION, LOCATION

It's true in real estate; it's also true in the GI microbiome. Where various species take up residence in the human GI tract has huge implications for your health and body shape.

As I've discussed, we have all lost numerous species in our GI microbiomes and acquired species that were foreign to our predecessors. But for many of us, the situation has become even worse. The colon, the most distal 4 to 5 feet of GI tract, is a section of intestine that is normally well adapted to housing fecal microbes. The high concentration of fecal species, rich with toxins, does not faze the colon that has, for instance, a thick protective layer of mucus that serves as a barrier between microbes and the intestinal wall. This is not to say that the colon is impervious to disruptive effects of the microbes it houses as such conditions as ulcerative colitis and colon cancer are increasingly looking like diseases that originate in a deranged colonic microbiome. But, with frightening frequency, a majority of modern people have had fecal microbial species ascend up into the 24 feet of small intestine where they don't belong: small intestinal bacterial overgrowth (SIBO). The three segments of small intestine—the duodenum, jejunum, and ileum—are not adapted to housing fecal microbial species, as the small intestine has evolved to be permeable and allow absorption of nutrients, such as vitamins, minerals, amino acids, and fatty acids, and lacks the protections against fecal microbes that the colon has. When trillions of fecal microbes come to inhabit the small intestine, they live and die at breathtaking speed, as microbes measure their lifetimes in hours, not years like us. When they die, fecal microbes release their toxins, especially a component of their cell walls called lipopolysaccharide endotoxin, which crosses the permeable small intestinal wall and enters the bloodstream, a process labeled "endotoxemia."

Should you ever experience an episode of bacterial sepsis in which bacteria invade the bloodstream, you might experience shock that requires the administration of intravenous medications to support your falling blood pressure, mechanical ventilation to keep you breathing during respiratory failure, and sometimes dialysis to compensate for failing kidneys, a dire situation in which the level of endotoxin in your bloodstream can be a hundredfold higher than normal, threatening your survival. There is no question that high levels of bacterial endotoxin in the bloodstream underlie critical human illness, sometimes enough to kill you. The level of endotoxemia that results from the invasion of fecal microbes into your small intestine does not reach the degree of that caused by critical illness but reaches a level higher than normal, posing chronic yet not acute threats to your health.

In less critical endotoxemia that develops from the invasion of fecal microbes into your small intestine, the blood levels of endotoxin are

200–400 percent higher than usual, not as high as in sepsis but enough to trigger numerous abnormal health conditions. This phenomenon, suspected as "leaky gut" by the alternative health community for many years, was formally validated in 2007 by a Belgian research group, corroborated many times since.[3] It handily explains how and why, for instance, the excessive proliferation of such fecal microbial species as *E. coli*, *Salmonella*, and *Campylobacter* can be experienced on the skin as rosacea or psoriasis, in the brain as depression or anxiety or cognitive impairment, in the heart as a heart attack or atrial fibrillation, in the thyroid gland as Hashimoto's thyroiditis, in muscle and joints as fibromyalgia or restless leg syndrome—no organ or body system is immune to the effects of bacterial breakdown products originating in the GI tract.

You can appreciate that this should cause us to reconsider *all* human health conditions as phenomena that result, at least in part, from the invasion of fecal microbes into the small intestine and the resultant endotoxemia. Without factoring in the contribution of disrupted bowel flora and endotoxemia, we cannot expect to have full control over the health conditions that surround us. As discussed in Chapter 5, this fundamental and disruptive process is far from rare but affects 50 percent or more of the population. And if you are dealing with weight and shape issues, it is likely to be more toward 100 percent and you are thereby exposed to increased risk, not just for distortions of shape but of numerous health struggles.[4] That's the bad news. The good news is that once you recognize these issues, you can be pointed in the direction of effective solutions that do not require doctors, pharmaceuticals, or hospital procedures.

But how can the lumps, bumps, and bulges that you are trying to manage be addressed through the GI microbiome? Overgrowth of fecal microbes in the colon or, worse, invasion of the small intestine by fecal microbes is a major driver of distorted body shape and size. You may have blamed moral weakness or faulty genetics, but much of the blame lies in the trillions of microbes occupying the GI tract. There are a number of ways in which these errant fecal microbes can expand abdominal fat, weaken and erode muscle, and wreak other forms of havoc on your body and its contours. Among the ways that microscopic creatures in your GI tract can ruin your day by generating distortions of shape and body composition include:

- Increased insulin resistance—You now know that this fundamental metabolic disruption increases accumulation of abdominal fat and blocks weight loss. A disrupted GI microbiome is one of the most powerful drivers of this effect.[3] Increased levels of cortisol triggered by insulin resistance also make matters worse.
- Increased inflammation—This goes hand in hand with insulin resistance. When abdominal fat expands, it provokes greater inflammation. Insulin resistance and inflammation drive abdominal fat accumulation that, in turn, increases insulin resistance and inflammation that further drive abdominal fat, around and around in a vicious cycle. You don't stop this process with calorie cutting or pharmaceuticals, but you do with strategies to address a disrupted GI microbiome.
- Loss of GI microbial species that produce butyrate—Recall that the fatty acid butyrate, produced by beneficial GI microbes, reduces insulin resistance and inflammation, thereby facilitating loss of abdominal fat while also yielding numerous beneficial effects such as reduced blood sugar and blood pressure, better sleep, and better GI health.[5]
- Loss of *Lactobacillus reuteri*—Remember that this unique microbial species plays two critical roles in determining body shape: (1) provoking the release of oxytocin from the brain, the hormone of body shape; and (2) taking up residence in the small intestine and producing bacteriocins, natural antibiotics effective in killing invading fecal microbes and thereby reducing endotoxemia. Restoring this microbe, lost by nearly everyone due to antibiotics and other factors, restores control over abdominal fat, weight, and muscle, with potential effects greater than anything I have ever before witnessed.
- Loss of *Lactobacillus gasseri*—*L. gasseri* is yet another microbial species that, like *L. reuteri*, has been reduced or eliminated

due to its susceptibility to antibiotics and other factors. Like *L. reuteri*, *L. gasseri* has the capacity to colonize the small intestine and produce bacteriocins, helping eradicate invading fecal microbes and thereby reducing endotoxemia.[6]

- Lack of *Bacillus coagulans*—This microbe is a bit different from the two aforementioned *Lactobacillus* species, in that it does not colonize the small intestine for any length of time but germinates from its spore-forming quiescent mode provided by fermented foods to become active in the small intestine where, like its two *Lactobacillus* friends, it produces potent bacteriocins. The advantage of *B. coagulans* is that it's also a wonderful factor in promoting regain of lost muscle.[7-9]

Informed management of the microbes dwelling in the tubular structure that begins at the mouth and ends at the orifice you wipe after a bowel movement can be magnificently powerful. Don't fall for overly simplistic conversations that say that this or that probiotic is effective or ineffective. Instead, we are going to work to rebuild a GI microbiome that more closely resembles that of the hunter-gatherers, yielding many of the same body-shaping benefits that they enjoy.

To make these concepts and strategies as easy as possible to adopt, I liken the GI microbiome to a backyard garden. I introduced this concept in my book *Super Gut*; it has proved to be such a helpful way to frame how we rebuild a healthy microbiome that I'd like to put this analogy to work once again.

HARVEST TIME

If you were determined to grow your own vegetables and fruit in place of the tasteless, nutrient-poor versions sold in most supermarkets, how would you accomplish this? Home gardeners all know that you start by preparing the soil, planting seeds, then watering and fertilizing throughout the growing season. Apply these efforts and you will harvest a bounty of tomatoes, cucumbers, and whatever else you planted.

I use this analogy because growing a healthy, bountiful, body shape–rebuilding GI microbiome is really not that different. You will not have to save seeds from a prior harvest or weed the soil, but many of the same principles that go into backyard gardening apply to the garden that is your GI microbiome.

Prepare the "Soil" of Your GI Microbiome

You start by laying out a section of land, say, a 10 × 10–foot area, clearing out sticks, stones, and weeds. You erect a barrier of wooden stakes or chicken wire to keep the rabbits, deer, and other creatures from consuming the fruits of your labor.

For the "garden" that is your GI microbiome, we begin with efforts to keep the "vermin" away, factors that are capable of disrupting your gardening efforts. I began this conversation in Chapter 5, where I discussed how excessive reliance on antibiotics, many of which are unnecessary, played a significant role in decimating your GI microbiomes. But let's review these and other factors from a GI microbiome perspective. You wouldn't, for instance, plant your garden in soil where you discarded unused turpentine, motor oil, or other chemicals. From the perspective of the GI microbiome, this means that you:

- Avoid food preservatives—Food preservatives kill microbes in food and also kill microbes in you. We therefore avoid foods with such ingredients as potassium sorbate, sodium benzoate, and the hundreds—*hundreds*—of others. Don't even try to memorize the list. If an ingredient sounds chemical, then it is and avoid. And remember: The best foods are those that lack an ingredient label.
- Banish synthetic sweeteners—While natural noncaloric sweeteners, such as monk fruit, stevia, and allulose are safe, the synthetic noncaloric sweeteners aspartame, neotame, saccharine, and sucralose wreak havoc on the microbiome composition of your GI tract, blocking your weight-loss and body-reshaping efforts, and should be avoided entirely.[10]

- Avoid foods that increase intestinal permeability—namely, wheat and other grains. The gliadin protein of wheat and related proteins of other grains are known to increase intestinal permeability, allowing microbial breakdown products to enter the bloodstream: endotoxemia. From prior discussions, you already know that this increases insulin resistance and inflammation and their effects that expand abdominal fat and reduce muscle.[11] The combination, by the way, of SIBO and the gliadin protein of wheat is an especially lethal combination, a duo that conspires to cause or worsen numerous common health conditions including expansion of abdominal fat. We therefore banish all wheat and grains.

- Filter drinking water—This is a strategy that reduces the dispersal of the intestinal mucus barrier by chlorine and chloramine that disrupts the microbial composition of the GI tract.

- Avoid pharmaceuticals that disrupt the GI microbiome—We therefore always question the need for a prescribed antibiotic, avoid stomach acid–blocking drugs, and avoid nonsteroidal anti-inflammatory drugs, such as ibuprofen and naproxen, which also disrupt the GI microbiome. There are likely hundreds of other pharmaceuticals that exert disruptive effects on the GI microbiome but, because the FDA does not require pharmaceutical companies to explore this issue prior to drug approval, we are largely in the dark on the effects of most pharmaceuticals on the microbiome.[12] But know that, by engaging in the strategies articulated in these pages, you are engaging in a process that frees you from reliance on numerous prescription drugs.

- Restore nutrients that play important roles in providing a nourishing environment for proliferation of healthy GI microbes—This is a list that is now familiar to you: vitamin D, iodine, magnesium, omega-3 fatty acids, and such nutrients as prebiotic fibers and hyaluronic acid that contribute to the strength of the intestinal barrier and allow the normal transit of digested food material through the GI tract.

Addressing the aforementioned factors begins the process of allowing beneficial microbes to reproduce and produce metabolites that add to your body-reshaping efforts. Just as it is important to take steps to safeguard your backyard garden, so it is to remove the factors that prevent or block your efforts to allow healthy microbes to proliferate in your GI tract.

Now that you've taken steps to prepare the "soil" of your GI microbiome garden, let's discuss how you plant the "seeds" of beneficial organisms.

Planting "Seeds" in Your GI Microbiome

These are the "seeds" of microbes that support our body-reshaping efforts. This is an evolving concept as we come to appreciate the unique roles that various microbes play. But we start by planting seeds for the most important GI microbes of all:

Lactobacillus reuteri—I cannot overstate the health and body-shaping effects the restoration of this one microbe provides. Recall that *L. reuteri*, especially when restored in high numbers (e.g., 300 billion per ½-cup serving of the "yogurt" that I shall show you how to make), helps you selectively target loss of abdominal visceral fat while also increasing muscle mass. It is not unusual, for instance, if you go to the gym to use the strength-training machines, to see your leg press increase from 200 pounds for ten repetitions to 300 pounds within a few weeks. Regaining that much strength and muscle provides significant advantages in reshaping your body. Restoring *L. reuteri* is also the start of your battle to push back SIBO, the flood of fecal microbes that have invaded the 24 feet of small intestine and thereby amplify insulin resistance.

Lactobacillus gasseri—This microbial species is the master of bacteriocin production, natural antibiotics effective against fecal microbes. Because, like *L. reuteri*, *L. gasseri* also takes up residence in the small intestine as well as the colon; the combination of the two microbes represents a powerful force in eradicating or preventing small intestinal colonization by invading fecal microbes. Human clinical studies in which abdominal visceral fat was measured using cross-sectional abdominal CT or MRI scans with *L. gasseri* alone have revealed marked reductions of visceral fat, reducing, for instance, abdominal visceral fat area by an impressive 21.6 cm², reflected by reductions in waist circumference.[13,14] Counts of *L. gasseri* achieving these effects were no more than 10 billion per day; we are going to exceed this number a minimum of tenfold to ensure big effects. It also makes among the most rich, thick, and delicious "yogurt" when fermented by itself. (Once again, it is not really yogurt, but something that looks and smells like yogurt.)

Bacillus coagulans—*B. coagulans* is a spore-forming species: that is, a microbe that enters a quiescent seedlike form that allows it to survive under harsh conditions. When ingested orally, it germinates in the small intestine where, like *L. reuteri* and *L. gasseri*, it produces bacteriocins that kill fecal microbes.[7] It also has unique effects on muscle and joints, reducing muscle injury incurred during strenuous work or exercise while also increasing muscle mass.

VICTORY IN THE BATTLE FOR YOUR SMALL INTESTINE

You may not be aware of it, but there has been a battle going on right below your diaphragm, a microbial battle for control of your small intestine.

As I've discussed, in an astounding proportion of people, the 24 feet of duodenum, jejunum, and ileum has been taken over by fecal microbes, species that belong in the colon and should stay in the colon, a situation labeled SIBO. In SIBO, the small intestine is dominated by pathogenic fecal species, such as *E. coli*, *Salmonella*, and *Campylobacter*—species commonly responsible for urinary tract infections, wound infections, and sepsis, as well as food poisoning from fecal contamination of food or water. As discussed in Chapter 5, you can recognize this situation if you have food intolerances or evidence of fat malabsorption, have any of the conditions highly associated with SIBO, such as fibromyalgia or irritable bowel syndrome, or test positive for hydrogen gas on the breath (we'll discuss this shortly).

But we have a secret weapon—restore microbes that most people lack or have lost: *L. reuteri, L. gasseri,* and *B. coagulans.* You could take them as probiotics, but we are going to take it a step further to amplify your hopes of taking back control over your small intestine and thereby factors that shape your body. We are going to ferment these microbes (allow them to proliferate) and *increase their number a hundred- or even thousandfold,* to ensure that they win the battle.

Say you're a general in an ancient army about to go to war against a force 10,000 soldiers strong. Would you rather bring 1,000 of your own soldiers to the battlefield or 100,000 to overwhelm the enemy? It's the same here: You are going to bring plenty of fighting personnel to this battle to overpower those nasty fecal microbes that have invaded your small intestine. I call the fermented combination of all three microbes "SIBO Yogurt" because I have been witnessing unprecedented success in normalizing SIBO (as measured by hydrogen breath testing). My team and I have run numerous flow cytometry measures (a method of counting microbes) on the yogurts that yield around 300 billion counts (colony-forming units [CFUs], a way of counting live microbes) per ½-cup (120 ml) serving. Compare that to the few billion usually provided by commercial probiotics.

HOW TO MAKE SIBO YOGURT

Here is how we put three microbial species to work in your small intestine, the battlefield for SIBO. While I call it SIBO Yogurt, I could have also called it Keystone Microbe-Restoring Yogurt since we are restoring species that you have lost but should have had throughout your lifetime. While we get started as SIBO Yogurt, it is perfectly fine, even preferable, to make a habit of at least intermittent consumption long after you have conquered SIBO.

To ferment these microbes, you will need:
- Some method of maintaining the mixture at around 100°F. A yogurt maker, sous vide (stick or basin), or Instant Pot

with a yogurt setting are the most popular choices. A note of caution: Some yogurt makers and Instant Pots have pre-set temperatures that can be too high. The two *Lactobacillus* species die at a temperature of 110°F or higher. You can run your device (with or without water in the basin, depending on your device) and insert a thermometer to measure the temperature. If the temperature is too high (ideally, no higher than 106°F) and the device does not allow you to adjust the temperature, you will need an alternative device. (See Appendix B for recommended devices.)

- Inulin powder—Fibers that feed the microbes during fermentation for a thicker end result and increased microbial counts.
- Microbes—You can co-ferment all three microbes together, in which case consider a somewhat higher temperature to accommodate the *B. coagulans* that "likes" higher temperatures but not so high that you kill the other two. You will need one capsule to start for each species. (See Appendix B for suggested commercial sources.) Because we can't control the relative numbers of each microbe with subsequent batches, consider starting from scratch after five or six batches. Alternatively, some people prefer to know that they are obtaining full counts of each microbe, in which case you can ferment them individually. If you do, the two *Lactobacillus* species should be fermented at 100°F, but the *B. coagulans* should be fermented at 115°F.
- One quart of organic half-and-half, whole milk, or cream. Be sure that there are no additives, such as gellan or xanthan gum, as they increase separation into curds (solid) and whey (liquid). I prefer half-and-half as it yields the best thickness and texture and remember: We never limit fat.

If co-fermenting all three together, follow these steps:

1. In a large glass or ceramic bowl, spoon in 1 tablespoon of inulin or raw potato starch.

2. Empty the contents of each probiotic capsule into the mixture.
3. Add 2 to 3 tablespoons of dairy and stir thoroughly. Break up any clumps with the spoon.
4. Add the remaining dairy and stir.
5. Cover and maintain at 100°F for 36 hours.

If fermenting each microbe individually, follow the same process in three bowls, using the fermenting temperatures as previously discussed.

For eradication of SIBO, consume ½ cup once per day of the three-microbe yogurt, or around ¼ cup of each individual-species yogurt, for a minimum of four weeks, longer for severe cases. If you would like to test breath hydrogen (H_2) to assess whether you have normalized this measure, you will have to stop consuming the yogurt for two weeks, then test. This is because *L. reuteri* is among the microbes that normally colonize the small intestine and converts fibers to hydrogen gas, giving the appearance of persistent SIBO.

If you do not have SIBO, or would like to maximize the benefits of one of these three microbes—such as increased muscle, increased libido, deeper sleep, smoother skin, and reduced skin wrinkles with *L. reuteri*—you can, of course, also ferment just this microbe alone to obtain the 300 billion counts that result with fermentation of this single species.

The combination of these three microbes as SIBO Yogurt is powerful. When I first combined all three as fermented "yogurt," I was surprised to see the majority of people eradicating SIBO, as documented by normalization of breath hydrogen. (See A Breath of Fresh AIRE: H_2 Testing for SIBO, page 189.) I was surprised because even a conventional antibiotic, such as rifaximin, the drug of choice to eradicate SIBO, has a track record of success of only 55–60 percent, and it's expensive, not covered by insurance, and shares the side effects of other antibiotics. Having something that resembles yogurt is therefore a benign but surprisingly effective method to banish fecal microbes from the small intestine.

Kathy, 68

"I HAVE SUFFERED WITH DIGESTIVE ISSUES MOST OF MY adult life. I took lots of antibiotics and ibuprofen over the years. I saw 8+ doctors and the only thing they did was prescribe antacid meds, send me to gastroenterologists to have endoscopies and colonoscopies, finding nothing wrong, and then shake their heads. I even had one doc tell me it was from having too many birthdays (meaning I was old and prone to problems).

"In 2005, I started seeing a naturopath and she had me taking lots of various supplements, and some of them did help, but I was still plagued with acid reflux, stomach pains, diarrhea, anxiety, and lots of body aches and pains. She did determine that I had a gluten intolerance, and once I stopped eating gluten, some of my symptoms got better but didn't totally resolve.

"Fast-forward to January 2020, I had major stomach pains that landed me in the emergency room, and after lots of tests, still nothing found. I was only able to eat broth, some meat, and green beans for about 2 months.

"I then adopted Dr. Davis's microbiome strategies, including learning about the yogurt treatment for SIBO. At first, I could only tolerate eating it for a week and would have to stop for a week, due to severe die-off symptoms. I kept at it until little by little my die-off symptoms eased up and I was able to eat it for longer periods of time. I purchased the AIRE device so I could do my own testing. It took me almost 2 years to get rid of SIBO, and every now and then it rears its ugly head and I go back to eating the yogurt until my symptoms resolve. I also learned about fermented foods, and with the introduction of that along with the SIBO Yogurt, my digestion and quality of life is so, so much better!

"SIBO Yogurt has been a miraculous treatment and so easy to make and eat."

————

If you test positive for SIBO by H_2 testing, or if you are comfortable proceeding empirically (i.e., based on your best judgment), then it is best to start with a minimum four-week course of the SIBO Yogurt. If you believe that you have an especially bad case of SIBO due to, for instance, a history of multiple food intolerances, severe bloating and diarrhea, having been exposed to multiple courses of antibiotics, and so on, there is no harm with a longer period of daily consumption. An occasional person requires months of consumption before H_2 breath normalizes. Because SIBO Yogurt provides important keystone species that have beneficial effects in rebuilding a healthy GI microbiome, as well as preventing the return of fecal microbes into the small intestine, it is a good practice to consume either the three microbes of SIBO Yogurt, or at least the *L. reuteri* Yogurt fermented alone, several times per week, even after breath H_2 has normalized or other signs of SIBO have receded. Until we figure out how to make these microbes take up permanent residence, we continue to replenish our GI tracts with these important species.

A BREATH OF FRESH AIRE: H_2 TESTING FOR SIBO

If you are among the 50 percent of Americans with this unnatural condition, then freeing yourself from the grip of misplaced fecal microbes can be life-changing. As discussed in Chapter 5, study after study has documented the high prevalence of SIBO in obesity, type 2 diabetes, irritable bowel syndrome, inflammatory bowel diseases, autoimmune diseases, fibromyalgia, restless leg syndrome, sleep apnea, fatty liver, and numerous other conditions. If you have a food intolerance to, say, prebiotic fibers, FODMAPs (fermentable oligo-, di-, monosaccharides, and polyols, which essentially are fibers and sugars), nightshades, histamine-containing foods, nuts, eggs or other foods, you can be confident that the underlying cause is SIBO and that correcting it nearly always frees you from the food intolerance. Because I am proposing that many cases of SIBO can be corrected by consuming SIBO Yogurt, an exceptionally benign method, it is reasonable, if you have one of the aforementioned conditions that are highly associated with SIBO, to proceed with the SIBO Yogurt even if you are not 100 percent certain that you have it. If I had said something like "We need to surgically remove a portion of your small intestine," then you should insist on knowing with certainty whether this is true or not. But if the solution is a homemade mixture that looks and smells like yogurt that you can make in your kitchen, absolute certainty is not necessary. And the microbial species being replenished by the SIBO Yogurt represent keystone beneficial species that nearly everyone has lost and yield spectacular benefits *even if SIBO is not present*: smoother skin, restored youthful musculature, increased libido, and deeper sleep among them.

You also have the option of testing for hydrogen (H_2) gas on the breath to identify SIBO, since many microbes produce H_2 gas but you cannot. You can have your doctor send you to a lab or clinic to test your breath for H_2 gas, a process that requires about four hours and costs several hundred dollars per test (several tests are typically needed). There is also the Trio-Smart test, for which you mail in your breath samples and they will be tested for hydrogen, methane, and hydrogen sulfide, which provides a wider assessment of abnormal microbial GI composition. You have the option of testing in the comfort of your kitchen with a consumer device that costs $150 to $200, the AIRE device. The current version tests for H_2 and methane gases and has the added advantage of being able to be used over and over again without additional charge. Breath testing in a lab or clinic, or with the Trio-Smart test, will yield results in days to weeks. The AIRE device yields immediate results, with values provided via the smartphone app that pairs with the device. (See Appendix C that lists resources for these tests.)

H_2 testing can be confusing for many people. Think of breath testing as a *mapping tool* that helps you locate where in the GI tract microbes are located; that is, are they in the colon where they belong, or are they in the small intestine where they do not? Never test at random times as you cannot distinguish normal H_2 production from microbes in the colon from abnormal small intestinal production of H_2. You are interested in knowing whether H_2 gas is produced soon (within 90 minutes) after prebiotic fiber is ingested before it has a chance to reach the colon.

Testing efforts begin with a diet absent of fibers and sugars for the preceding twelve or more hours: no legumes, root vegetables, onions, garlic, fruit, and no alcohol; only meats, oils, and green leafy vegetables. On the morning of testing, obtain a baseline level before breakfast, then ingest 2 teaspoons of inulin powder (a prebiotic fiber metabolized by most microbes, beneficial and harmful) in coffee, tea, or any other food. (A meal with foods of your choosing at this point will not interfere with testing.) You then retest for breath H_2 every 30 to 45 minutes for up to 90 minutes. On the AIRE device, any rise in H_2 (on a scale of 0 to 10) of four or more units (corresponding to 20 parts per million [ppm] if performed in a lab or clinic; each AIRE unit = 5 ppm) represents a positive test for SIBO. A positive reading after 90 minutes could be ileal SIBO (SIBO far down the small intestine in the ileum) or could be normal H_2 production from microbes in the colon. If you obtain an indeterminate reading of, say, a rise from 1.2 to 8.6 that occurs at 120 minutes, use your judgment on whether this represents SIBO or not.

AIRE testing for methane gas, useful to identify overgrowth of methane-producing species that cause constipation, is positive with any rise of two units, equivalent to 10 ppm on the other testing platforms. The rules for interpretation

of hydrogen sulfide gas (from Trio-Smart or a testing laboratory) have not yet been worked out, but consider this test if
unexplained diarrhea is an issue. If you test positive for H₂ or
methane, most people enjoy success in reducing these factors
just by taking the steps detailed here—SIBO Yogurt, prebiotic
fibers, consuming fermented foods, etc.—that help rebuild a
healthy GI microbiome.

Another important aspect of planting "seeds" in your garden of
bowel flora is to include plenty of fermented foods in your lifestyle.
These are tomatoes, onions, garlic cloves, radishes, cabbage, sliced
cucumbers, and other foods that you allow microbes to feed on for
days to weeks before consuming. Although this was a common practice
up until your great-grandparents' day, it has been largely abandoned
by most modern people, especially in the United States. (Many people in parts of Europe and Asia have maintained this practice, a likely
explanation for the reduced incidence of many diseases, including obesity and heart disease, that prevail in these populations.)

Fermented foods, such as sauerkraut or kimchi, provide microbes
to your GI tract. We ferment foods by relying on microbes naturally
resident on the surface of, say, cabbage or cucumbers, or you can
use sources of microbes, such as a starter culture you purchase. (See
Appendix B for fermentation basics.) You can also use commercially
fermented foods that contain live microbes. For instance, purchase
a commercial sauerkraut or fermented pickles (making sure it says
"naturally fermented" or "contains live cultures," or some equivalent
phrase, to make sure that it is indeed fermented), take a couple of
tablespoons of the liquid from this commercial product, add to your
mix of brine and vegetables, and the microbes passed on will do the job
for you.

Emerging science tells us that the microbes responsible for fermentation of food, such bacterial species as *Leuconostoc mesenteroides*,

Pediococcus pentosaceus, and *Weisella*, and fungal species, such as *Saccharomyces boulardii*, do not take up residence in the human GI tract but simply pass through. But in their journey through the GI tract, they provide nutrients or metabolites that nourish important species living in that GI tract, increasing their populations and their production of metabolites that benefit health, an example of what microbiologists call "cross-feeding."[15] Inclusion of fermented foods thereby yields a long list of benefits, including influencing your shape and body composition. This phenomenon is one of the most helpful strategies you can follow that increases the diversity of microbes dwelling in your GI tract while also protecting you from unhealthy species. One of the most powerful fermented foods can be obtained from my recipe for sparkling fruit juices that uses the fungal species *S. boulardii*. Although we avoid fruit juices in general, due to excessive sugar content, when you ferment juices, the microbes consume the sugars, leaving little to none at time of consumption when done properly. And you will have fruit-flavored sparkling sodas to enjoy that help cultivate diversity in bowel flora and limit the damage to your GI microbiome during a course of antibiotics.

Please don't confuse what I am calling "yogurt" here with the products you find on supermarket shelves—they are two entirely different things. We begin with microbial species with specific properties, such as bacteriocin production or provoking oxytocin release, then ferment for prolonged periods to obtain high counts of microbes. This is distinct from store-bought products that employ microbes with little beneficial effects, ferment for brief periods (typically 6 to 12 hours), and thereby yield far lower bacterial counts, and often contain added sugar, high-fructose corn syrup, thickening agents, synthetic colorings and flavorings—many of the factors we are trying to avoid. I call our fermented projects, such as SIBO Yogurt "yogurt," but they're not really yogurt. They look and smell much like yogurt, but they are distinct and unique. Many in my community call our yogurts "progurts" or "nogurts."

The basics of fermenting foods, including *S. boulardii* sparkling juices, can be found in Appendix B.

WATER AND FERTILIZE YOUR MICROBIOME GARDEN

There's no need to gather up some cow manure or composted table scraps to feed your "garden" of bowel flora. But just as you harvest the greatest bounty of produce at the end of the growing season if you water and fertilize your backyard garden, so will you enjoy the greatest bounty of healthy microbes in your GI tract (and other body parts, interestingly) by properly feeding them.

In addition to the metabolites provided by ingesting fermented foods, you can add further by ingesting fibers, polysaccharides, and other factors that nourish important microbial species, such as *Akkermansia*, *Faecalibacterium*, and *Lachnospiraceae*, key microbes that facilitate loss of abdominal visceral fat and support regain of muscle. "Water and fertilize" these microbes, and they will provide many nice functions for you that include:

- Compete with pathogens—such as the microbes of food poisoning, fecal microbes, and the dreaded *C. difficile* that can result after a course of antibiotics.[16]
- Produce the fatty acid butyrate that nourishes intestinal cells and enters the bloodstream to exert effects such as reduced blood glucose, reduced insulin resistance, reduced blood pressure, improved sleep, healthier skin, and reduced abdominal fat.
- Produce vitamins B_1, B_2, B_3, B_5, B_6, B_9 (folate), B_{12}, and K_2. In other words, many of the nutrients that people obtain via nutritional supplements should really be obtained from GI microbes.[17]
- Consume problematic metabolites—such as oxalates and uric acid. The fact that microbes have enormous power in reducing such factors suggests that the tough diet restrictions and pharmaceuticals introduced to manage these health issues are really misguided efforts that ignored the contribution of the microbiome.[18,19]
- Play a large role in mental and emotional health—It has become clear that GI microbes, largely via the so-called gut-brain axis,

play important roles in what goes on in your brain, the emotions you experience, your internal dialogues. The boost in oxytocin that results from restoration of *L. reuteri*, for example, is communicated through the vagus nerve up from the GI tract to the brain, thereby generating feelings of love, empathy, and generosity. The reduction in endotoxemia that results from watering and fertilizing your GI microbiome reduces the microbial contribution to anxiety, anger, stress, depression, and suicidal thoughts.[20]

• Mediate hormonal effects—A disrupted GI microbiome can cause low testosterone that makes men passive or lose interest in sex, increases estrogen that distorts male physiology and increases risk for breast cancer in females, prevents conversion of the T4 thyroid hormone (e.g., as provided by taking levothyroxine thyroid tablets) to the active T3, causing persistent symptoms of hypothyroidism. Oxytocin, cortisol, and growth hormone are among the other hormones influenced by the GI microbiome with substantial effects on abdominal fat and muscle.[21,22] The fiber content of your diet therefore plays a major role in overall hormonal health.

As you can appreciate, these are not subtle or minor effects but large, often dramatic, effects, all exerted via the microscopic creatures dwelling in your GI tract. We therefore need to properly feed and nourish this world of microbial species.

The factors that feed our microbes take on a number of forms, a topic of ongoing debate among biochemists on how to label them. We do not need to get bogged down with this biochemical debate. The husband-and-wife microbiologist research team at Stanford, Drs. Erica and Justin Sonnenburg, suggest that we conveniently combine the various designations of these factors that feed microbes under one umbrella term: microbiota-accessible carbohydrates (MACs). While even this broader designation does not include all factors that nourish microbes, it comes close. All MACs share the property of being resistant to human digestion: You ingest them, but you lack the digestive enzymes to break them down. Microbes in your GI tract, however, possess those enzymes, yielding nutrients that "fertilize" beneficial microbial species.[15]

MACs that "water and fertilize" your GI microbes originate with various plant foods that include:

- Root vegetables—onions, garlic, shallots, leeks, asparagus, radishes, daikon radish, beets, turnips, Brussels sprouts, carrots, ginger, fennel, celeriac, rutabaga, white potatoes (raw only)
- Legumes—black, white, kidney, lima, and pinto beans; chickpeas, hummus; peas; lentils
- Mushrooms—button, portobello, shiitake, oyster, morel, chanterelle, lion's mane, and many others
- Chia seeds, flaxseeds—These foods provide a combination of MACs, as well as "bulking" fibers that can be helpful if loose stools are a struggle for you.
- Nuts—walnuts, pecans, almonds, pistachios, hazelnuts
- Fruit—MACs are concentrated in the peel and rinds, not so much the pulp
- Green bananas and plantains—This is a unique source that some prefer to add to their smoothies. Unripe, these plants are green and essentially inedible. So add them to smoothies by cutting lengthwise, removing their skins, then chopping coarsely before adding to a blender.
- Shirataki noodles—These noodles made from a root, very low in net carbs, are rich in the MAC glucomannan.

For convenience, many MACs, including inulin, acacia fiber, and galactooligosaccharide, are commercially available as powders or as mixtures. See the section Recipes to Support Your Battle of the Bulge (pages 201–233), which provides tasty ways to be sure prebiotic fibers and related compounds are part of your daily habits.

To ensure an ideal daily intake, I suggest that you include a source of MACs *with every meal*. For instance, add a teaspoon or two of inulin to your cup of morning coffee or tea (4 to 8 grams MAC). Add 2 table-spoons of black beans to your morning omelet (2 grams MACs) along with some chopped onions and garlic (2 grams MACs). Finely cube half a medium-size raw white potato to toss into your green salad (10 grams MACs) along with a small sliced onion (4 grams MACs) and several sliced white mushrooms (2 grams MACs). Add a handful of raw mixed nuts (unquantified MACs) and you have easily topped your 20-gram goal to cultivate healthy bowel flora that support your body-reshaping goals. (See Appendix B for a list of the MAC content of various foods.)

One very important fiber, unlike nearly all other fibers that are sourced from plants, is hyaluronic acid, which I discussed earlier. Despite being sourced from animal products, especially organs and skin, it is an important fiber MAC that exerts substantial effects in small amounts, such as 100 mg (0.1 grams). Hyaluronic acid, being a compound that adds to moisture and structural integrity of organs such as skin and joints, can only be sourced from animal products, since there are no plant sources of this MAC. As most people do not want to add organ meats to their daily routine, hyaluronic acid is available as a nutritional supplement in powder or capsule form.

Also, don't be misled by online conversations stating that if you bake a potato, then allow it to cool, the original fibers that were converted into sugars by heating will return to their original fiber state, a process called retrogradation. The quantity of sugar that reverts back to fiber is so small as to be inconsequential, leaving that cooled potato as nearly all sugar. The only form of potato we consume for our purposes are therefore raw white potatoes.[23]

We remain mindful of net carbs as we only desire the benefits of the MACs that nourish microbes but do not want to provoke excessive quantities of blood glucose, insulin, and glycation that impair our body-shaping and youth-preserving efforts. For this reason, you may notice that some root vegetables are not listed, such as sweet potatoes or yams, as they provide only a small amount of fiber but excessive amounts of sugar when cooked, and even when raw (in contrast to white potatoes). You can include them, but know that you can exceed our 15-gram net carb limit quite readily, with 22 grams net carbs per cooked medium-size sweet potato, for example.

Is there an ideal intake of MACs per day? Most evidence suggests that 20 grams or more daily generates maximum beneficial effect.[24] It's not that hard to achieve, especially if you follow my advice to include at least one MAC-containing food in every meal. Variety is also key, as taking in a variety of different MACs helps cultivate a wide variety of beneficial microbes.

Please don't be guilty of neglecting your intake of MACs as this can have unhealthy long-term consequences. Neglecting MAC intake can lead to an impaired intestinal mucus barrier; increased endotoxemia; excessive proliferation of mucus-consuming species, such as *Akkermansia*; excessive proliferation of bile acid–tolerant species that add to risk for colon cancer; expansion of abdominal fat; and erosion of muscle. Take care of your "garden" of bowel flora, and it will pay you back in dividends many times over. Not only will you have better bowel health, but better sleep; better moods and attitudes; more youthful skin; youthful libido; and, yes, better body contours, pushing you closer and closer to a flat, muscled abdomen; lithe and beautiful arms, shoulders, and thighs; and being freed of all the useless concerns that plague people who subscribe to conventional and ineffective ways of living.

IS THERE ANY ROLE FOR PROBIOTICS?

Too often, people embrace commercial probiotics as the sole solution to their microbiome struggles. But I mention probiotics last because of all the strategies I've discussed, probiotics are the *least* helpful. They can have a role but not the starring role that many expect. The shortcomings of current commercial probiotics include:

- Haphazard formulation—Nearly all probiotics are random collections of microbes with no attention to "collaborations" via metabolites, so-called cross-feeding.
- Failure to include keystone species—Because such species as L. reuteri and L. gasseri are foundational, that is, they

support the proliferation of numerous other species, it is a mistake to not include at least a few such keystone species. Including keystone species means that the benefits of the probiotic are much greater.

- Low bacterial counts—If a product contains 10 billion CFUs per capsule spread out among twenty species, that means that there are 500 million microbes of that species in each capsule—sounds like a lot, but in the world of microbes it is a trivial number. One of the reasons that counts are kept low is to keep costs low, as microbes can be very expensive. (You can appreciate that our yogurts and other ferments are a low-cost way to amplify bacterial numbers dramatically.)
- Failure to include small intestinal colonizing species—since this is where SIBO occurs.
- Failure to include species/strains known to produce bacteriocins—especially those with effects against fecal microbes.
- Introducing strategies that delay release of microbes— Some companies put their microbes into a capsule designed to delay release into the colon, thereby losing the benefits of small intestinal release. We do not want delayed release.

Probiotic formulation remains a work in progress. The probiotic of the future will likely address all the aforementioned issues while also adding important microbes that are not yet available. You will see, for instance, such species as *Faecalibacterium prausnitzii*, *Lachnospiraceae*, and *Clostridia butyricum* play a role in future formulations.

In the meantime, tend your garden of bowel flora by adopting my discussed strategies, and view commercial probiotics as providing modest additional advantage—if any—but not the sole strategy that can cause you to neglect all the other factors that provide greater benefits. See Appendix B for the handful of recommended probiotic products.

THE AGE OF THE MICROBIOME

In this chapter, we've considered all the strategies that you can adopt—or, more correctly, readopt the lost lifestyle practices of preceding generations—to rebuild something that more closely resembles a healthy microbiome that supports your efforts to manage weight, the distribution of fat, and the restoration of muscle, as well as favorably affect other aspects of health. Even though the microbiome has been with us in some form for as long as our species has walked the planet, this is a chapter that could not have been written only a few years ago. That's how fast knowledge and understanding of the microbiome has progressed.

Insights into the power of consuming fermented foods and fibers that nourish microbes, restoration of microbial species that colonize the small intestine, and species that participate in the gut-brain axis were unimaginable as recently as when former president Barack Obama took office, or in 2007 when Apple released its first iPhone. It means that you have access to a tool set to reclaim control over multiple aspects of health that your mom and dad didn't have. And because it requires a generation or two for conventional practicing physicians to embrace new science, it also means you have access to cutting-edge insights that have not even begun to enlighten your neighborhood doctor.

Combine microbiome insights with other new strategies in diet, nutrient replacement, and restoring factors lost due to blundering dietary guidelines, and you have a powerful collection of ways to accomplish all your ambitions in enjoying a youthful body shape and composition.

RECIPES TO SUPPORT YOUR
BATTLE OF THE BULGE

Here are recipes designed to augment the effects you are working toward by following *SUPER Body* strategies. These dishes will help you stay on track in obtaining beneficial microbes, prebiotic fibers and related compounds, collagen, hyaluronic acid, and carotenoids, all adding to your body-reshaping efforts.

I am mindful of price in following these recipes, especially costs associated with purchasing microbes for fermentation. I've included some inexpensive ways to ferment microbes by starting with commercially available products. For example, you can make kombucha simply by buying commercial kombucha and fermenting juices or teas with it.

To maximize benefits, it really helps to include at least one serving of a fermented food and one serving of a food containing MAC or prebiotic fiber *in every meal*. It's not that tough. Take a sip, for instance, of *S. boulardii* or *B. subtilis* sparkling juice, and a teaspoon of inulin powder in your morning coffee. Make a habit of including a small serving of a legume or root vegetable in every meal. The more you engage in including these foods in your daily routine, the easier it gets and the greater the benefits. The recipes included here will get you started.

All recipes provide serving sizes that keep your net carb intake at or below our 15-gram net limit. And, of course, you will find no mention of wheat, grains, gluten-free processed flours, corn oil, or other unwanted food ingredients.

PROBIOTIC AND PREBIOTIC RECIPES

L. REUTERI YOGURT

L. reuteri is the first microbe I chose to ferment and play around with. By sheer dumb luck, I chose what is probably the number one most important microbe for shape, body composition, and numerous other aspects of health. Obtaining *L. reuteri* daily, or at least several times per week, should therefore be the cornerstone of all your efforts.

The method I use for making *L. reuteri* yogurts serves as a prototype for how to make many other yogurts starting with other *Lactobacillus* and *Bifidobacteria* species. In other words, use the same temperature and fermentation time for most other fermenting species.

Note: If you would like to avoid dairy and use coconut milk (canned) instead, follow these additional steps to prevent separation in the final result:

- Choose a coconut milk with no additives (e.g., gellan gum or xanthan gum). Guar gum is okay.
- Preheat the coconut milk to 180°F for several minutes, then allow to cool to <100°F.
- Add 1 teaspoon of guar gum.
- Blend with a stick blender for at least 1 minute.
- Add a microbe source *after* blending.

MAKES 8 SERVINGS

L. reuteri source (See Appendix B for recommended sources.)
1 tablespoon inulin powder
1 quart organic half-and-half

Empty the contents of one *L. reuteri* capsule or packet into a large bowl.

Add the inulin, followed by 1 to 2 tablespoons of the half-and-half. Stir until mixed, breaking up any clumps.

Add the remainder of the half-and-half and mix.

Cover and maintain at 100°F for 36 hours.

SIBO YOGURT

To ferment these three microbes together, we need to make allowances for the higher fermenting temperature of the *B. coagulans* that reproduces best at 115° to 122°F, a temperature that kills *L. reuteri* and *L. gasseri*. We can compromise by using a temperature of 106°F, higher to make *B. coagulans* "happy" but not high enough to kill the other two temperature-sensitive species. Once again, we ferment for 36 hours to maximize the microbial numbers. If you'd prefer to avoid dairy, see the *L. reuteri* Yogurt recipe (page 202) for the additional steps required to use coconut milk.

MAKES 8 SERVINGS

Sources of *L. reuteri*, *L. gasseri*, and *B. coagulans* (See Appendix B
   for recommended sources of microbes.)
1 tablespoon inulin powder
1 quart organic half-and-half

Empty the contents of each microbial source capsule or packet into a large bowl.

Add the inulin, followed by 1 to 2 tablespoons of the half-and-half. Stir until mixed.

Add the remainder of the half-and-half and mix, breaking up any clumps.

Cover and maintain at 106°F for 36 hours.

SACCHAROMYCES BOULARDII SPARKLING JUICE

Here's a delightful way to rebuild a healthy GI microbiome using sparkling juices. Although juices start with high quantities of sugar, the process of fungal and bacterial fermentation reduces sugars to negligible levels.

S. boulardii is a fungal species, a close relative of *S. cerevisiae* that is used to make wine and beer but better adapted to inhabiting the human GI tract. While it is labeled a "probiotic," it is really more like a prebiotic, providing nutrients to bacteria to feed and nourish them. *S. boulardii* is especially helpful in protecting your GI microbiome during and after a course of antibiotics. By fermenting, you will create delicious sparkling sodas that can be wildly effervescent. Juices have a lot of sugar, so we ferment to not just maximize fungal counts but also minimize sugar content, as *S. boulardii* vigorously metabolizes sugar. The end results should be non- or minimally sweet. Juices can be diluted, if desired, by adding filtered or distilled water after the completion of fermentation.

By fermenting, you will be increasing microbial counts and thereby benefits while enjoying delicious effervescent, nonsugary juices. Consume ¼ to ½ cup at least once per day, more frequently if taken during a course of antibiotics.

MAKES 4 TO 8 SERVINGS

1 capsule *S. boulardii* CNCM I-745 probiotic (e.g., Florastor brand, which is widely available), or ¼ cup Health-Ade brand kombucha

1 quart juice without preservatives (e.g., no potassium sorbate or sodium benzoate)

Empty the contents of the probiotic capsule into the juice, cap, and lightly agitate. Loosen the cap—very important, as you will see carbon dioxide bubbles forming after 24 hours that if capped too tightly can literally cause the container to explode. Alternatively, you can purchase venting caps at a beer brewing store; these cost a few dollars. Allow to sit on your kitchen counter for around 60 hours. Taste—if still sweet, allow to ferment for an additional 12 hours, or until minimal sweetness remains.

BACILLUS SUBTILIS SPARKLING JUICE

As with the *Saccharomyces boulardii* Sparkling Juice (page 204), we again put fermentation to work, this time with the bacterial species *B. subtilis* that, like *S. boulardii*, generates effervescence while consuming sugars down to negligible levels.

B. *subtilis* is a spore-forming microbe that germinates in the small intestine and produces potent bacteriocins. While body-reshaping benefits of this microbe are not as powerful as those provided by *L. reuteri*, *B. subtilis* adds further advantage in reducing insulin resistance and abdominal fat while increasing muscle mass. It is worth making consumption of *Bacillus subtilis* Sparkling Juice a routine part of your everyday habits.

If you have an Aldi grocery store near you, it should carry a kombucha product from VitaLife that is an inexpensive source of this important microbe. Alternatively, a product from GT (a popular brand of kombucha), called Agua de Kefir, is another source of this bacterial species. If sourced elsewhere, look for the DE111 strain as this strain is a vigorous producer of carbon dioxide to generate effervescence.

MAKES 4 TO 8 SERVINGS

1 capsule *B. subtilis* probiotic (minimum 2 billion CFUs), or
  ¼ cup VitaLife Kombucha or GT Agua de Kefir
1 quart juice without preservatives (e.g., no potassium sorbate
  or sodium benzoate)

Empty the contents of the probiotic capsule into the juice, cap, and lightly agitate. Loosen the cap—very important, as you will see carbon dioxide bubbles forming after 24 hours that if capped too tightly can literally cause the container to explode. Alternatively, you can purchase venting caps at a beer brewing store; these cost a few dollars. Ferment at 90°F for 60 hours, or until no longer sweet. If residual sweetness persists, allow to ferment for an additional 12 hours, or until minimal sweetness remains.

KEY LIME CHEESECAKE PREBIOTIC SHAKE

Here, one shake supplies a whopping 20 grams of prebiotic fiber that stacks the odds in favor of reducing insulin resistance and thereby adding to your body-reshaping efforts.

Net carbs for this shake are around 4 grams, well below our cutoff of 15 grams. Also, this shake provides a good opportunity to add ½ cup of your choice of yogurt—e.g., *L. reuteri, L. gasseri,* or *B. coagulans.* Either stir in the yogurt with a spoon or pulse minimally in a blender so that bacteria are not destroyed by vigorous blending.

If budget permits, choose organic potatoes.

MAKES 1 SHAKE (ABOUT 12 OUNCES)

1 medium-size raw white potato, chopped coarsely
2 ounces (¼ cup) cream cheese, at room temperature
¼ cup Key lime juice
Sweetener equivalent to 2 tablespoons sugar (see pages 246–247)
½ teaspoon pure vanilla extract
½ cup water
½ cup yogurt (optional; see headnote)

Combine the potato, cream cheese, Key lime juice, sweetener, vanilla, and water in a blender and blend until smooth. If adding yogurt, add to the mixture and pulse briefly or mix with a spoon. Serve.

CHOCOLATE-COVERED CHERRY SMOOTHIE

Here's a tasty way to combine collagen peptides, the beneficial microbe *Lactobacillus plantarum*, and prebiotic fibers to obtain multiple beneficial effects. The taste is reminiscent of chocolate-covered cherry candies.

L. plantarum is another interesting microbe that adds further to body-reshaping benefits, helping reduce abdominal fat and build muscle. It also provides many other beneficial effects, including improved skin health and appearance.

Each serving of this smoothie adds 20 grams of collagen to your day, the dose shown to exert advantageous body-shaping, skin, and joint benefits.

To make this recipe easier, purchase frozen cherries with their pits removed. Note that the cherries will need to be fermented for 24 hours before making this smoothie. You could also ferment more than the 1 cup in the recipe, reserving the additional amount for future use. The Good-Belly juice used as a source for *L. plantarum* is widely available in most major supermarkets and big-box stores (usually in the dairy refrigerator). Or you could, of course, purchase this microbe as a probiotic capsule, also widely available. Recall that, by fermenting, you increase the number of microbes and thereby increase body-reshaping and other benefits.

MAKES 2 SERVINGS

1 cup cherries (pits removed)
¼ cup GoodBelly brand juice
1 (13.5-ounce) can coconut milk
4 level tablespoons collagen peptides
1 teaspoon inulin or other prebiotic fiber
2 tablespoons unsweetened cocoa powder
Choice of sweetener equivalent to 3 tablespoons of sugar
    (see pages 246–247)

Puree the cherries in a blender. Transfer to your fermenting vessel, add the GoodBelly juice, stir, and cover. Place in your choice of fermenting device set to 90°F for 24 hours.

After completing fermentation, uncover and add the coconut milk, collagen, inulin, cocoa powder, and sweetener, and shake or stir until thoroughly mixed and all clumps have dissolved.

NO-BAKE PROBIOTIC RASPBERRY CHEESECAKE

And you thought you'd be deprived following this lifestyle?! Here, we convert an unhealthy, indulgent, sugary dessert into a delicious healthy treat, complete with a probiotic microbial species that helps shrink your waist, *Lactobacillus gasseri*, champion keystone species, small intestinal colonizer, and bacteriocin producer.

If you haven't yet fermented *L. gasseri*, follow the same method used to make *L. reuteri* Yogurt (page 202) but use the starter probiotic specified in Appendix B.

MAKES 8 SERVINGS

CRUST:

> Coconut oil, avocado oil, or unsalted butter, for the pan
> 1½ cups ground pecans, walnuts, or almonds
> 3 tablespoons unsalted butter, melted
> 1 teaspoon unsweetened cocoa powder
> Pinch of sea salt

FILLING:

> 2 (8-ounce) bricks cream cheese, at room temperature
> ½ cup *L. gasseri* yogurt
> Sweetener equivalent to 1 cup sugar (see pages 246–247)
> 1 teaspoon pure vanilla extract
> Juice of ½ lemon
> 1 cup heavy cream
> 1 cup fresh or frozen raspberries

Make the crust: Grease a 9-inch pie pan with the coconut oil. Combine the ground nuts, butter, cocoa powder, and salt in a medium-size bowl, and mix thoroughly. Transfer the mixture to the prepared pie pan and, using a wet spoon, press along the bottom and partially up the sides. Set aside.

Make the filling: Combine the cream cheese, yogurt, sweetener, vanilla, and lemon juice in a large bowl, and mix thoroughly.

In a separate bowl, whip the cream until stiff peaks form. Pour the whipped cream into the cream cheese mixture and gently mix by hand. Pour the mixture into the piecrust.

Refrigerate for a minimum of 8 hours. Arrange the raspberries around the edge before serving.

ONE-MINUTE FROZEN STRAWBERRY PROBIOTIC YOGURT

Our probiotic yogurts make delicious frozen yogurts. Don't worry: Freezing does not kill the microbes. Although strawberries are specified here, any other frozen berries work equally well.

MAKES 2 SERVINGS

1 cup frozen strawberries
Sweetener equivalent to 2 tablespoons sugar
    (see pages 246–247)
1 cup your choice of yogurt (*L. reuteri*, *L. gasseri*, or *L. crispatus*
    are good choices)

Pulse the berries in a blender until they are fragmented. Add the sweetener and yogurt, and pulse briefly until the yogurt solidifies. (We avoid vigorous blending to minimize killing the yogurt microbes.)

ASPARAGUS AND MUSHROOM PIZZA

Think of pizza as a vehicle for prebiotic and carotenoid-rich foods. Here, asparagus, onions, garlic, and mushrooms provide a variety of prebiotic fibers and related compounds, along with carotenoid-rich tomato paste (300% higher carotenoid content than tomato or pizza sauce) and kale.

MAKES 6 SERVINGS

PIZZA CRUST

> 8 ounces cream cheese
> 1 cup shredded mozzarella cheese
> ¼ cup water
> ¾ cup almond flour
> ½ teaspoon sea salt

TOPPINGS

> 4 tablespoons extra-virgin olive oil
> 1 yellow onion, diced
> 2 garlic cloves, minced
> 4 ounces white mushrooms, sliced
> 4 ounces asparagus, chopped
> 4 ounces kale, torn or cut into small pieces
> Sea salt and freshly ground black pepper
> 1 (6-ounce) can tomato paste
> Sweetener equivalent to 2 teaspoons sugar (see pages 246–247)
> 1 cup shredded mozzarella cheese

Preheat the oven to 350°F. Line a baking sheet or pizza pan with parchment paper.

Make the crust: Combine the cream cheese, mozzarella, and water in a medium-size microwave-safe bowl, then microwave in 30-second increments until the cheeses are melted, stirring slightly with each return to the microwave. Add the almond flour and salt and stir thoroughly.

Place the dough on the prepared pan and, with moistened hands or a spoon, press into a 12-inch circle, repeating with wet hands or spoon as needed. Form a raised outer edge all around the dough. Bake for 15 minutes, or until just starting to brown. Remove from the oven and set aside.

Make the toppings: Heat 2 tablespoons of the oil in a large skillet over medium-high heat. Add the onion and garlic and cook, stirring frequently, for 5 to 6 minutes, or until the onion becomes translucent. Add the mushrooms, asparagus, kale, and salt and pepper to taste, and cook, stirring frequently, until all the vegetables are softened.

Combine the tomato paste, remaining 2 tablespoons of olive oil, and the sweetener in a small bowl and stir until mixed. Spread over the pizza crust with a spatula, then distribute the mozzarella on top, followed by the vegetable mixture. Return the pizza to the oven for an additional 10 minutes, or until the cheese has melted.

FETTUCCINE WITH ROASTED RED PEPPER TOMATO SAUCE

Hearts of palm pastas have become my pasta replacement of choice lately, as this is a form of noodle that provides prebiotic fiber effects on GI microbes similar to inulin. This dish is also bursting with carotenoid content since we use tomato paste (300% greater carotenoid content than tomato sauce) and roasted red peppers.

MAKES 4 SERVINGS

3 tablespoons extra-virgin olive oil
1 yellow onion, diced
3 to 4 garlic cloves, minced
1 (8-ounce) jar roasted red peppers, drained
1 (6-ounce) can tomato paste
½ teaspoon dried oregano
1 cup water
Sea salt and freshly ground black pepper
2 (12-ounce) packages hearts of palm fettuccine noodles
Parmesan cheese (optional)
Fresh basil leaves (optional)

Heat the oil in a large skillet over medium heat, then add the onion and garlic and cook until the onion is translucent, for 5 to 6 minutes. Meanwhile, puree the red peppers in a food chopper or food processor; stir into the onion mixture, followed by the tomato paste, oregano, water, and salt and black pepper to taste. Set aside.

Bring 2 cups of water to a boil in a medium-size saucepan over high heat. Lower the heat to maintain a gentle boil. Add all the noodles, cover, and cook, stirring occasionally, until they are softened, for about 5 minutes. Drain the noodles in a colander. Serve topped with the sauce mixture. Optionally, serve with grated Parmesan cheese and finely chopped fresh basil leaves.

L. REUTERI COLESLAW

This recipe was inspired by my friend and prolific cookbook author Dana Carpender, who, among her many talents, loves to concoct clever recipes for this microbe.

I specify *L. reuteri* for this recipe, but you can substitute other *Lactobacillus* or *Bifidobacteria* species to make the yogurt that serves as the basis for this healthy coleslaw. *L. brevis* and *L. crispatus*, for example, make delicious yogurts that are perfect for this coleslaw recipe.

Shredded raw potato is included in the ingredients, an easy way to up your intake of prebiotic fibers.

MAKES 8 SERVINGS

1 tablespoon apple cider vinegar
½ cup *L. reuteri* (or other) Yogurt (page 202)
½ cup mayonnaise (preferably a brand made with avocado or
    light olive oil rather than soybean or canola)
½ cup peeled and shredded raw white potato
1 tablespoon prepared yellow mustard
1 teaspoon dried onion powder
Sweetener equivalent to 1 tablespoon sugar (see pages 246–247)
Sea salt
1 head cabbage (about 1 pound), chopped finely, or 1 bag
    preshredded

Combine the apple cider vinegar, yogurt, mayonnaise, potato, mustard, onion powder, sweetener, and salt to taste in a large bowl and mix. Toss the cabbage in the mixture to coat.

PROBIOTIC RANCH DRESSING

My original Wheat Belly Ranch Dressing has been a perennial hit among my readers. So here it is again, this time with a probiotic twist.

MAKES ABOUT 2 CUPS

1 cup yogurt (*L. reuteri, L. gasseri, L. crispatus* are good choices)
½ cup mayonnaise (preferably a brand made with avocado or
    light olive oil rather than soybean or canola)
1 tablespoon white wine vinegar
½ cup grated Parmesan cheese
1 teaspoon garlic powder or finely minced garlic
1½ teaspoons onion powder
Pinch of sea salt

Mix the yogurt, mayonnaise, and white wine vinegar in a medium-size bowl. Stir in the Parmesan, garlic powder, onion powder, and salt. Add nonchlorinated water, 1 tablespoon at a time, if you desire a thinner dressing. Store in an airtight container in the refrigerator for up to 4 weeks.

PROBIOTIC VEGGIE DIP

Here is another way to put our favorite *L. reuteri* Yogurt (page 202), with its exceptional tanginess, to work: as a dip for fresh vegetables. Include fresh-cut veggies on a charcuterie board (see recipe, page 219) to dunk into this dip or my Probiotic Ranch Dressing (above), alongside fermented meats, olives, and cheeses, for a feast of body-reshaping foods and microbes.

MAKES ABOUT 1½ CUPS

1 cup mayonnaise (preferably a brand made with avocado or
    light olive oil rather than soybean or canola)
½ cup *L. reuteri* Yogurt (page 202)
Juice of ½ lemon
1 teaspoon onion powder

1 teaspoon garlic powder
½ teaspoon dried dill

Combine the mayonnaise, yogurt, lemon juice, onion powder, garlic powder, and dill in a small bowl and mix.

CREAM OF ASPARAGUS PREBIOTIC SOUP

Here's a dish that adds a significant quantity of prebiotic fibers for body-reshaping benefits.

MAKES 6 SERVINGS

½ cup extra-virgin olive oil or coconut oil
2 cloves garlic, minced
1 medium-size yellow onion, chopped
1 leek, rinsed well and sliced
2 cups coarsely chopped dandelion greens
4 cups chicken stock
1 pound asparagus, chopped coarsely
1 cup coconut milk
Sea salt and freshly ground black pepper

Heat the oil in a large skillet over medium-high heat, add the garlic and onion, and sauté for 5 to 6 minutes, stirring occasionally, until the onion becomes translucent. Add the leek, dandelion greens, chicken stock, and asparagus and cook, stirring frequently, until the greens wilt and asparagus softens. Add the coconut milk, plus salt and pepper to taste, then cover and cook for 5 minutes, stirring occasionally.

Remove from the heat, allow to cool down for 10 minutes, then transfer to a blender. Blend until liquefied, then serve. (Reheat, if desired.)

LENTIL SOUP

Lentils provide a source of the galactooligosaccharide variety of prebiotic fiber that, along with polysaccharides and prebiotic fibers from the mushrooms, onion, and garlic, makes a contribution to your body-reshaping efforts.

MAKES 6 SERVINGS

¼ cup extra-virgin olive oil
1 medium-size yellow onion, chopped
2 garlic cloves, minced
8 ounces white button mushrooms, sliced
1 teaspoon ground turmeric
1 teaspoon ground cumin
1 tablespoon curry powder
½ teaspoon ground nutmeg
1 (13.5-ounce) can coconut milk
4 cups chicken stock or water
1 cup dried red or yellow lentils
3 carrots, sliced
2 celery ribs, sliced
Sea salt and freshly ground black pepper

Heat the oil in a large saucepan over medium-high heat, then add the onion, garlic, mushrooms, turmeric, cumin, curry powder, and nutmeg. Cover and cook, stirring frequently, until the onion becomes translucent and the mushrooms are lightly browned, for 5 to 6 minutes. Remove from the heat and set aside.

Combine the coconut milk, chicken stock, lentils, carrots, and celery in a large saucepan over high heat. Bring to a boil, then lower the heat and simmer, covered, for 20 minutes, or until the lentils are tender. Stir in the onion mixture. Add salt and pepper to taste.

GINGER EGGPLANT

Here's a tasty way to add more prebiotic fibers from both ginger and eggplant, as well as the carotenoids of eggplant. If you are unable to locate Japanese eggplant, use standard eggplant, but be sure to slice it thinly.

SERVES 4

½ cup coconut oil
2 pounds Japanese eggplant, sliced thinly lengthwise
2 tablespoons roasted sesame oil
6 garlic cloves, minced
1 tablespoon minced fresh ginger
2 tablespoons sesame seeds
3 tablespoons tamari or gluten-free soy sauce

Heat ¼ cup of the coconut oil in a large skillet over medium-high heat, and add the eggplant, distributed in a single layer. The eggplant may need to be cooked in several batches to maintain a single layer. Turned when lightly browned, for 2 to 3 minutes per side. Transfer the cooked eggplant to a large bowl.

In the same skillet, heat the remaining ¼ cup of coconut oil over medium heat, then add the sesame oil, garlic, ginger, and sesame seeds. Stir frequently until the garlic has softened, for about 2 minutes. Pour the mixture into the bowl with the eggplant, add the tamari, and toss until mixed.

COLD RAMEN NOODLES

Shirataki noodles are an ultralow-carb form of noodle perfect for re-creating healthier Asian dishes that provide the unique glucomannan pre-biotic fiber. Add water chestnuts and bok choy for additional prebiotic fibers, and fermented fish sauce for probiotic bacterial species, and you have a wonderful and tasty light dish to serve with some riced cauliflower or hearts of palm rice.

MAKES 2 SERVINGS

2 (6-ounce) packages shirataki noodles
1 (12-ounce) can water chestnuts
1 cup finely chopped bok choy or spinach
2 teaspoons roasted sesame oil
1 teaspoon fermented fish sauce (e.g., Thai Kitchen brand)
2 tablespoons tamari or gluten-free soy sauce
2 teaspoons onion powder
1 tablespoon sesame seeds

Place the shirataki noodles in a colander and rinse briefly. Transfer to a medium-size bowl and add the water chestnuts, bok choy, sesame oil, fish sauce, tamari, onion powder, and sesame seeds and mix.

L. REUTERI RADISH SALAD

Here is a variation on a high-carb potato salad that you will be proud to share at a summertime barbecue or picnic. Radishes and onions pro-vide fibers that nourish bowel flora while the yogurt dressing is another opportunity to increase your intake of body-reshaping L. reuteri. Add to its probiotic/fermented food content by including chopped pickles or other veggies that you have fermented.

MAKES 6 SERVINGS

4 cups radishes, quartered
4 hard-boiled eggs, sliced
1 cup finely chopped celery

1 red onion, minced

¾ cup *L. reuteri* Yogurt (page 202)

¾ cup mayonnaise (preferably a brand made with avocado or
   light olive oil rather than soybean or canola)

¼ cup prepared yellow mustard

2 teaspoons onion powder

1 tablespoon vinegar

¼ cup chopped fermented pickles

Sea salt

Bring about 1 quart of water to a boil in a large saucepan. Put in the
radishes and cook for 15 minutes. Drain and set aside to cool.

   Combine the eggs, celery, onion, yogurt, mayonnaise, mustard,
onion powder, vinegar, pickles, and salt to taste in a large bowl. Once
cooled, add the radishes and mix thoroughly.

PROBIOTIC CHARCUTERIE BOARD

This is not so much a recipe but a reminder that fermented meats are
another food to consider adding to your habits. Raw meats that are naturally fermented, such as sopressata, prosciutto, saucisson, pancetta, and
numerous ethnic varieties are a source of beneficial probiotic microbes.
(Don't confuse fermented meats with cured or processed meats made
with, for instance, sodium nitrite, which is regarded as a carcinogen. When
you purchase cured meats, make sure no sodium nitrite is listed on the
label. Unfortunately, in many human clinical studies, no distinction is
made between fermented meats and nitrite-cured meats, and they are
often misleadingly lumped together.)

   Charcuterie boards are also an opportunity to introduce fermented
cheeses. You'll need to distinguish cheese that is fermented from nonfermented by the more complex flavors and mention of aging in fermented
cheeses on the product label—such varieties as Roquefort, bleu, Gruyère,
Gouda, feta, and many others. These are the cheeses you're more likely to
find in the artisanal cheese refrigerator rather than in the dairy refrigerator next to milk and cream. Olives are another food to include, but it is not
always easy to distinguish fermented from nonfermented. As with cheese,

olives purchased in the artisanal cheese or olive bar are more likely to be fermented as compared to those in jars next to brined (not fermented) pickles.

Consider adding some fresh-cut vegetables to your charcuterie board; for example, celery sticks, jicama, radishes, or endive leaves to dip into Probiotic Ranch Dressing (page 214) or Probiotic Veggie Dip (page 214).

BAKED CHICKEN THIGHS WITH MUSHROOM SAUCE

This simple recipe is a reminder to get away from food stripped of nutritional value, such as boneless, skinless chicken breast. We choose chicken thighs here for the greater fat, collagen, and hyaluronic acid content, coupled with the polysaccharide fibers of mushrooms and the inulin prebiotic fiber of onions and garlic.

MAKES 4 SERVINGS

2 tablespoons extra-virgin olive or coconut oil
1 yellow onion, chopped
3 garlic cloves, minced
8 ounces white button mushrooms, sliced
4 ounces portobello mushrooms, sliced
½ cup coconut milk or heavy cream
¼ cup white wine
2 pounds chicken thighs
Sea salt and freshly ground black pepper

Preheat the oven to 375°F.

Heat the oil in a large skillet over medium heat, then add the onion and garlic. Cook, stirring frequently, until the onion is translucent, for about 5 minutes. Add the button and portobello mushrooms and cook, stirring occasionally, until they have softened, for 3 to 5 minutes. Stir in the coconut milk and wine. Remove from the heat and allow to cool for 5 minutes, then puree in a food chopper or food processor, reserving about one-quarter of the mushrooms. Add the reserved mushrooms to the pureed mixture.

Meanwhile, place the chicken thighs in a single layer in a baking pan, sprinkle with salt and pepper to taste, and bake for 45 minutes.

Serve the baked chicken topped with the mushroom sauce.

COLD CUCUMBER SOUP

I specify *Lactobacillus rhamnosus* in this recipe, useful for adding to your body-shaping and muscle-restoring effects, as well as being an important probiotic species. (*L. rhamnosus* GG strain is one of the few species shown to reduce the incidence of *Clostridium difficile* enterocolitis, for instance, which can develop after a course of antibiotics.) Because this is a cold, rather than usual hot, soup, we don't kill the microbes.

MAKES 2 SERVINGS

2 large cucumbers, sliced thinly
2 tablespoons extra-virgin olive oil
2 garlic cloves, minced
½ cup fresh mint, minced
1 teaspoon dried dill
1 cup *Lactobacillus rhamnosus* (or other) yogurt (page 202)
Juice of ½ lemon
Sea salt

Combine the cucumbers, olive oil, garlic, mint, and dill in a blender and blend until smooth. Stir in the yogurt (do not mechanically blend), lemon juice, and salt to taste. Optionally, refrigerate for 4 to 6 hours before serving.

PORK FRIED "RICE"

Pork fried rice has been among the favorite recipes I've provided in the past, but here it is reconfigured to increase prebiotic fiber and carotenoid content, to better contribute to your body-reshaping goals. We use hearts of palm "rice" that provides fibers to nourish gut microbes; cauliflower rice is another good choice.

MAKES 4 SERVINGS

4 tablespoons coconut oil
4 scallions, sliced
½ cup coarsely chopped roasted red peppers
2 garlic cloves, minced
2 large eggs, whisked
8 ounces pork tenderloin, cut into ½-inch cubes
¼ cup tamari or gluten-free soy sauce
2 (12-ounce) packages hearts of palm rice

Heat 2 tablespoons of the oil in a large skillet over medium-high heat, then add the scallions, peppers, garlic, and eggs; stir continuously until cooked through. Transfer the mixture to a bowl and set aside.

In the same pan over medium-high heat, cook the pork until no longer pink, for 5 to 7 minutes. Add the tamari and stir in the egg mixture and hearts of palm rice. Cook, stirring frequently, until the hearts of palm have softened, for about 3 minutes.

COLLAGEN AND HYALURONIC ACID RECIPES

Here are some great ways to include collagen peptides and hyaluronic acid in various dishes beyond just adding a scoop to a smoothie.

COLLAGEN-HYALURONIC ACID BROWNIES

Here's a tasty way to get your collagen in the form of chewy brownies. Choose chocolate with the least sugar, such as Lindt Excellence 90% Cocoa Supreme Dark Chocolate bars or Lily's Dark Chocolate Style Baking Chips.

MAKES 9 BROWNIES

Coconut or other oil, for the pan
½ cup collagen peptides
¼ teaspoon hyaluronic acid powder
½ cup unsweetened cocoa powder
1 cup almond flour
Sweetener equivalent to ½ cup sugar (see pages 246–247)
6 tablespoons unsalted butter, melted
2 ounces dark chocolate, melted
2 large eggs
½ cup coconut milk (canned)

Preheat the oven to 350°F. Oil an 8-inch square baking pan with coconut oil.

Combine the collagen peptides, hyaluronic acid, cocoa powder, almond flour, and sweetener in a large bowl and mix. Add the butter, chocolate, eggs, and coconut milk and mix thoroughly.

Pour the mixture into the prepared baking pan and bake for 45 minutes, or until a knife or toothpick inserted into the center comes out dry. Remove from the oven, allow to cool, then cut into brownies.

COLLAGEN MINUTE MUFFIN

Here's a quick and easy recipe for a collagen-rich muffin-in-a-mug that provides another way to include collagen in your daily routine. Top with a bit of whipped cream or dark chocolate shavings for added variety. Here, I specify strawberries, but any other variety of berry, cinnamon, and nutmeg, or even a savory cheese can be used.

One muffin provides around 20 grams of collagen.

MAKES 1 MUFFIN

3 level tablespoons collagen peptides
½ cup almond flour
1 tablespoon ground golden flaxseeds
2 tablespoons unsalted butter or coconut oil, melted
Sweetener equivalent to 2 tablespoons sugar
    (see pages 246–247)
½ cup fresh or frozen strawberries, chopped roughly
1 large egg
¼ cup water

Combine the collagen, almond flour, flaxseeds, butter, sweetener, berries, egg, and water in a large, microwave-safe mug and mix thoroughly.

Microwave on HIGH for 3½ minutes. Allow to cool for several minutes before consuming.

MOCHA MINT COLLAGEN KEFIR

Kefirs are among the richest sources of microbial species from a fermented food, which helps you rebuild a body-reshaping GI microbiome.

Use either commercial kefir or a kefir you made yourself starting with a bit of commercial kefir or kefir starter. (See how to make kefir in the recipe under The Basics of Room-Temperature Fermentation, page 226.)

MAKES 2 SERVINGS

2 cups kefir
1 teaspoon instant coffee granules
4 level tablespoons collagen peptides
¼ teaspoon hyaluronic acid
1 tablespoon unsweetened cocoa powder
½ teaspoon mint extract, or a small handful of fresh mint
    leaves, chopped finely
Sweetener equivalent to 1 tablespoon sugar
    (see pages 246–247)

Combine the kefir, coffee, collagen, hyaluronic acid, cocoa, mint, and sweetener in a shaker and shake until well mixed. Serve cold or at room temperature.

THE BASICS OF ROOM-TEMPERATURE FERMENTATION

It helps to break microbes that ferment foods into two categories: microbes that ferment best (i.e., achieve maximum reproductive rate, and thereby greatest microbial numbers) at human body temperature, and those that ferment best at room temperature. While there are exceptions to this categorization, most microbes of interest will fall into one or the other category. This concept will become useful when you venture out on your own to begin fermenting unique species not discussed here.

You will find the methods I use to ferment microbes at human body temperature in the recipes for *L. reuteri* Yogurt (page 202) and SIBO Yogurt (page 203). The "rules" for fermenting at human body temperature apply to nearly all microbes that fall under *Lactobacillus* and *Bifidobacteria* designations (genera). Here, let's discuss how to ferment microbes at room temperature, useful for fermenting vegetables and other foods.

Microbes that ferment at room temperature are typically naturally resident on the surface of vegetables that proliferate under the right conditions (saline, no or limited exposure to air room temperature). Alternatively, you can use a starter culture that accelerates the process (a list of suggested sources follows).

You will need a jar or ceramic vessel and a means of keeping veggies submerged beneath the surface of the brine, away from oxygen that inhibits fermentation. I use an old olive jar and a heavy drinking glass that fits into the mouth of the jar and keeps veggies submerged below the surface of the liquid; others use a small plate weighted down with a stone. You can buy a fermentation kit, but it's really simple to assemble your own with items you likely already have on hand.

- **Vegetables:** Raw onions, peppers, asparagus, cucumbers, radishes, garlic, carrots, cabbage, green beans, daikon radish, mushrooms, and others—any vegetable can be fermented. Chop the vegetables into bite-size pieces. Combine the vegetables to create unique flavors; for example, asparagus and onions or green beans and garlic.

- **Herbs and spices:** Peppercorns, dill, garlic cloves, coriander seeds, mustard seeds, caraway seeds, rosemary, oregano. Many people also add grape or berry leaves to increase crispiness.
- **Sea salt or other salt:** Use any salt except iodized salt (iodine kills microbes).
- **Water:** Use filtered water, spring water, or distilled water (i.e., water without chlorine or fluoride).

BASIC FERMENTATION

Fill a jar or fermentation vessel with water, then add salt until the water tastes lightly to moderately salty, typically 2 tablespoons per quart of water.

Add the vegetables and your choice of herbs or spices. Stir to mix the vegetables with the salt water and to release any trapped air bubbles.

Submerge the vegetables and cover them with a plate or other clean object to keep them below the surface, then cover the vessel to keep pests out. Alternatively, add additional water and/or vegetables to bring the water level to the very top of the vessel, leaving little to no air once the cap is applied. The system should not be airtight but only loosely covered because the process of fermentation produces gases that must be released.

Set the vessel aside for at least 3 days. The time required varies with the type of vegetables used and temperature, but fermentation can go on for weeks. As a rule of thumb, if you rely on the microbes naturally resident on the surface of a vegetable such as a cucumber or cabbage leaves, fermentation will require a minimum of 3 weeks. If you use a starter culture, fermentation time will be abbreviated to several days. Taste your ferment as it progresses. Once you obtain the flavor and texture you desire (a skill that you will acquire as your experience with fermentation grows), refrigerate the jar; this will slow further fermentation.

Optionally, after the vegetables have fermented, add ¼ cup of vinegar (white wine, red wine, apple cider, or other vinegar) per quart of fermented mixture to enhance the flavor.

Should any white or other colored growth appear on the top, this is mold; skim it off and discard. It does not harm the fermentation process, and your fermented foods will remain safe for consumption for at least 4 weeks in the refrigerator.

SUGGESTED STARTER CULTURE RESOURCES:

Cultures for Health: culturesforhealth.com

Oxiceutics*: oxiceutics.com

Positively Probiotic: positivelyprobiotic.com

Fermentaholics: fermentaholics.com

Commercial vegetables that are prefermented, such as sauerkraut, fermented pickles, fermented beets, apple cider vinegar, and kombucha (unpasteurized) can also be used as a starter. Just add a couple tablespoons of the liquid from the pickles, sauerkraut, or other fermented food to your brine mixture and proceed as described. Recipes for making kombucha from commercial kombucha and kefir from commercial kefir follow. Like using a commercial starter, this typically accelerates the fermentation process, with good results typically within several days.

*Dr. Davis has a consulting or other financial relationship with this source.

KOMBUCHA

Kombucha is traditionally made by obtaining a SCOBY (symbiotic collection of bacteria and yeast) from someone who has been fermenting this beverage, who may have received their original SCOBY from an elder family member. In some parts of the world, people are brewing kombucha that got its start generations ago.

A simple work-around that costs almost nothing is starting with a commercial kombucha. It won't have the same diversity of microbes as kombucha brewed from a SCOBY that has survived numerous generations, but it will nonetheless contain interesting microbes. And if you generate your own self-perpetuating kombucha, you never have to purchase a starter source again.

Start with a commercial kombucha, preferably one with multiple microbes that include the fungal species *Saccharomyces boulardii* and bacterial species *Bacillus coagulans* or *Bacillus subtilis*, as well as other bacterial species. The GT brand is my preferred starter (around $3.50 for a bottle), as it includes these microbes and is widely available in most major supermarkets and big-box stores. Alternatively, you could start with a commercial kombucha starter from one of the sources listed on page 228.

Green and black teas used to make kombucha provide their own collection of health benefits, such as cross-linking mucin proteins in intestinal mucus, converting mucus from a semiliquid barrier to a semigel and thereby affording better protection of your intestinal lining against bacterial toxins and adding to the benefits of reducing endotoxemia.

Don't panic when you see sugar listed in the ingredient list: The sugar is consumed by the microbes. The final product should contain little to no residual sugar. If you do detect some sweetness, allow to ferment on your kitchen counter for another 24 hours, or until the sweetness is gone. Unlike fermenting vegetables, there is no need to prevent exposure to air. You should, however, keep your kombucha covered with plastic wrap or some other cover.

MAKES 1 QUART

1 quart water (filtered or distilled)
3 green or black tea bags
¼ cup sugar

Bring the water to a boil in a medium-size saucepan, then turn off the heat. Place the tea bags in the water and steep for 3 to 5 minutes. Stir in the sugar.

Cover and set on a countertop or other dry area to ferment for a minimum of 7 days. Taste for sweetness: You want little to no residual sweetness. When the sweetness is at your desired level, pour the liquid through a strainer into a jar and refrigerate, leaving a few tablespoons of kombucha in the jar. (If you detect a lot of vinegar or alcohol, it means you fermented for too long, a process that typically requires 3 to 4 weeks or more.)

Top up the jar with another quart of tea and another ¼ cup of sugar, and repeat the previous process.

KEFIR

Just as with kombucha, you can start fermenting your own kefir starting with a commercial starter culture, some kefir that someone else has been making, or even some commercial kefir you purchased at a supermarket. You will quickly see that making your own kefir is so incredibly easy and that fermentation proceeds rapidly to generate a thick, rich end result. Should you replace the dairy milk with canned coconut milk, add 1 teaspoon of guar gum and 1 tablespoon of sugar to the mixture and ferment until no residual sweetness is present. As with kombucha, there is no need to prevent exposure to air, although your mixture should be covered.

MAKES 1 QUART

Kefir starter, or 2 tablespoons commercial kefir
1 quart whole milk

Add the kefir starter to the milk, agitate lightly, and set aside on your kitchen counter for 24 hours, then refrigerate.

HEALING LEMON GREEN TEA

This is an improvement on a recipe for Clove Green Tea, which was originally included in *Super Gut*, meant to facilitate healing of the GI tract.
Green tea catechins, a unique class of beneficial plant polyphenols, such
as epigallocatechin, cross-link the mucin proteins in intestinal mucus,
converting it from a semiliquid to a more protective semigel. Cloves provided the essential oil eugenol, which thickens the intestinal mucus lining, while inulin blooms *Faecalibacterium*, the most vigorous producer of
butyrate, which nourishes and heals the intestinal wall.

In this variation, we add some hyaluronic acid. Recall that hyaluronic
acid, even in small amounts, is a potent fiber that blooms numerous beneficial species in the GI microbiome, amplifying any effort to reshape body
contours. I added a squeeze of lemon juice to enhance palatability as the
clove component is somewhat strong.

I have found these teas to be most useful early in your program when
you may be dealing with severe colonic dysbiosis or SIBO. The mucus
effects of this combination are both soothing and protective.

MAKES 4 SERVINGS

>   2 cups filtered or distilled water
>   1 tablespoon whole cloves
>   2 green tea bags
>   2 teaspoons inulin powder
>   ⅛ teaspoon hyaluronic acid powder
>   Juice of ½ lemon

Bring the water to a boil in a small or medium-size saucepan, then
lower the heat to maintain a gentle boil. Add the cloves, cover, and
simmer for 10 minutes. Remove from the heat.

Pour the liquid through a strainer to remove the cloves. Add the
tea bags to the hot liquid and allow to steep for 3 to 5 minutes. Stir in
the inulin and hyaluronic acid, breaking up any clumps. Squeeze the
lemon juice into the mixture prior to serving.

FERMENTED TOMATOES, EGGPLANT, AND RED ONION

Here's a delightful mixture of vegetables that ferments well, since the sugar in tomatoes accelerates the fermentation process. I specify Japanese eggplant for its softer taste and thinner skin, but conventional eggplant can be substituted. If you use a commercial starter culture for vegetable fermentation or some of the liquid remaining from a commercially fermented product such as pickles or sauerkraut, you can expect to see fermentation proceed within 5 to 7 days. If you rely on the microbes normally resident on the surface, 3 to 4 weeks is typical. Get in the habit of tasting your ferments to gauge whether they have achieved the flavors and textures you desire.

Of course, this is just one example of fermented vegetables, a mixture of prebiotic fiber sources (eggplant, onions, garlic) and carotenoids (eggplant, tomatoes). There are numerous other variations: baby onions, scallions, radishes, mushrooms, garlic cloves, leeks, daikon, and so on. Add fresh rosemary, basil, oregano, bay leaves, peppercorns, mustard seeds, and other herbs and spices to vary flavors.

Remember, your fermentation setup should allow no contact of air with the brine and veggies. Once your mixture has fermented and achieved the taste and texture you prefer, it is no longer necessary to prevent the veggie-air interface and you can refrigerate the veggies to slow or stop the fermentation.

MAKES 1 QUART

1 quart brine (filtered or distilled water to which 2 tablespoons non-iodized salt has been added)

2 to 3 small Japanese eggplants, cut into ½-inch cubes

1 cup cherry tomatoes, halved

1 red onion, quartered and sliced

4 to 5 garlic cloves, halved

2 to 3 tablespoons roughly torn or chopped fresh basil

1 tablespoon peppercorns

1 tablespoon mustard seeds

1 teaspoon dried dill seeds, or 1 sprig fresh dill

Fill your fermenting vessel with the brine, then add the eggplants, tomatoes, red onion, garlic cloves, basil, peppercorns, mustard seeds, and dill seeds. You may have to add more brine so that the setup you use does not allow submerged veggies to contact air.

FERMENTED SALSA

Here's how to make fermented salsa from scratch. The tomatoes are very fermentation-friendly, yielding fermented salsa within a few days. You can save time and effort by using a commercial salsa, but just be sure that the brand you choose contains no preservatives or emulsifying agents.

If making from scratch, be sure to choose ripe, flavorful tomatoes. Consider adding jalapeño or other pepper for added hotness.

MAKES 16 OUNCES

    2 cups coarsely chopped fresh tomatoes
    1 red onion, chopped
    2 tablespoons fresh cilantro
    2 garlic cloves
    Juice of 1 lime
    Sea salt and freshly ground black pepper

Combine the tomatoes, onion, cilantro, garlic, and lime juice in a food processor, food chopper, or blender, then pulse until the desired consistency is obtained. Add salt and pepper to taste.

To ferment, use a starter culture or the juice left over from pickles, sauerkraut, or other vegetable fermentation. Place in your fermentation setup for a minimum of 3 days.

AFTERWORD

I N *SUPER BODY*, WE'VE DRAWN LESSONS FROM A NUMBER OF unconnected sources. We've examined the emerging science of the microbiome that, like the exploding world of artificial intelligence, is providing a flood of new ideas and strategies at a rate so rapid that a day doesn't pass in which some new and powerful revelation isn't reported. We've drawn lessons from the exceptionally powerful phenomenon of the wisdom of crowds provided by this chaotic but powerful tool called social media—often flawed and filled with potholes but, when used properly, can yield empowering feedback and insights into unexpected sources of new information. We've drawn from anthropological insights obtained by studying the record of how our species has survived and adapted against incredible odds over the millennia. We all live in a unique time in human history, a time in which all these sources of knowledge are providing better answers to so many previously unanswered questions. I cringe to think just how ignorant we were on issues of health just as recently as when the first edition of the US Dietary Guidelines for Americans was released or the first drug for reducing cholesterol hit the market. Our understanding of health, nutrition, and shape and body composition was as primitive and ignorant as believing that cigarettes were good for lung health or that women were ill-equipped to vote—absurd and shameless. Yes, that would properly describe the last century of nutritional advice, weight loss, and an understanding of human health.

We should therefore take lessons from the blunders committed over the last several decades by consensus "wisdom" in the guise of dietary guidelines or advice on how to lose weight. We need to step back and recognize that much of what we hear and see relevant to health, nutrition, and body composition is shaped by marketing, persuading us to buy products and services that benefit a company or industry. Is there really any intrinsic human need for corn chips or breakfast cereal? If we conducted our lives in ways that are consistent with our genetic heritage, would there be any need for Wegovy or gastric bypass? Would products like Spanx or a procedure like liposuction have any place in our efforts to look better?

Let's face it: No one wants to have a protuberant abdomen, flabby arms, or double chin. You just want to be slender, youthfully muscled, and glowing with health and vigor—none of which is achievable with an injectable drug, surgical procedure, or conventional notions of diet.

Despite all the lessons learned, there are still millions of people who are willing to spend thousands of dollars on pharmaceuticals or bariatric procedures to regain youthful body contours. But for these millions, regaining youthful contours is an increasingly unreachable goal as the root causes of the various lumps, bumps, and bulges plaguing modern people simply remain unaddressed. Distortions of weight and body shape are now even afflicting youth: obese seven-year-olds, fourteen-year-olds with type 2 diabetes, teenagers injecting themselves with the newest GLP-1 agonist drug or undergoing gastric bypass. Make no mistake: The health toll, physical and emotional, of these phenomena are staggering, the worst in human history, yet they continue to be endorsed by most physicians and others in health care. Even as recently as the 1950s or '60s, it would have been unimaginable to think that you needed the assistance of a pharmaceutical to fit into a size 4 dress or 32-inch-waist pants, or to subject children to surgical procedures to reduce stomach volume.

Don't make the approach detailed in *SUPER Body* harder than it should be. During the first week, you are simply readopting the diet of our ancestors, though allowing for some modern conveniences. It is actually a lot easier in our time than it was in theirs, as you no longer have to hunt or forage, nor are you exposed to pro-longed periods of deprivation due to drought, flood, winter, or war. During the second week, you reintroduce nutrients that you should have obtained naturally. Again, your efforts are small compared to the search for fresh water, killing and consuming the organs of land ani-mals, catching fish, and foraging for wild plants—you can just visit the grocery store or health-food store, or order online with a few clicks, not risking attack by wild predators or falling from a tree or tumbling down a cliff. The third week is admittedly more challenging than our ancestors had it. You are, after all, engaging in something that our ances-tors didn't understand or recognize but managed unknowingly: the microbiome. But by taking steps to address this incredible universe of microbes that can be restored to your body, you are gaining advan-tages that your doctor, dentist, or dietitian simply doesn't know how to provide.

Recognize that the ideas promoted here address natural, physio-logic needs written into your genetic code, addressing factors that our species acquired over thousands of generations. The diet we adopt is similar to that followed in 50,000 BC. The nutrients we supplement were all obtained effortlessly by drinking water, eating wild plants, hunting animals for meat and organs, and exposing ourselves to sun-light. And by participating in the incredible experience called the microbiome that we share with all living creatures and the environ-ment, we restore the lush and varied collection of microbial species that support our health and body contours. But we've abandoned so many of these natural sources that we need to compensate, to circum-vent all the problems such as those in modern food and water, to obtain all the factors that we require, needs written into our genetic code.

You should be able to run your hands along a flat, muscled abdo-men. You should be able to ascend stairs or a hill, bounding up at rapid speed, regardless of how many decades you've walked this earth. You should be able to lift your children or grandchildren up high in the air, celebrating this incredible phenomenon called human life, unimpaired and unencumbered by the distortions of shape and body composition caused by the misinformation of the last several decades. Open your eyes to the wisdom of our planet and species, and you can become enlightened to the ways that the world really works.

The world, when properly interpreted and implemented, works in your favor. It's only when misinterpretation, misrepresentation, and profit-seeking motives enter the equation that just living your life leads to health problems and distortions of body shape. It's an odd conundrum: Rejection of modern advice opens the door to regaining control over shape and body composition, as well as happiness, contentment, satisfaction, love, empathy, generosity, and looking incredible in a bathing suit.

APPENDIX A
DIET RESOURCES

DIET SUMMARY

Here's a detailed summary of dos and don'ts in crafting your natural body-reshaping program. Recall that we preferentially chose whole foods over processed or ultraprocessed foods. A slice of beef, a three-egg omelet with mushrooms and peppers, or an avocado would qualify, for example, while a box of breakfast cereal, a "tart" you pop in the toaster, french fries, or frozen pizza would not.

Take advantage of condiments that liven up food. Keep a supply of horseradish, wasabi, and mustards (Dijon, brown, Chinese, Creole, chipotle, wasabi, horseradish, and regional mustards), and look for ketchups with no added sugar or high-fructose corn syrup. Tapenades (spreads made of a paste of olives, capers, artichokes, portobello mushrooms, and roasted garlic) can be purchased ready-made to spare you the effort and are wonderful toppings for eggplant, eggs, chicken, or fish. Salsas, of course, are available in a wide variety or can be readily made in minutes, using a food processor. (These are examples of processed foods in which the basic structure and ingredients have not been altered but remain largely intact.) Always check the label on such products to be sure no preservatives or thickening agents have been added.

Explore seasonings and spices beyond salt and pepper. Herbs and spices, such as basil, oregano, rosemary, cinnamon, cumin, nutmeg, turmeric, various dried chile peppers (e.g., ancho, chipotle), and dozens of other herbs and spices are available, fresh or dried, in any well-stocked grocery store.

In the world of grain-like foods, or "pseudograins," two stand apart as they don't share the excessive carbohydrate exposure of quinoa or buckwheat: These are flaxseeds and ground psyllium husk. Use ground flaxseeds as a hot cereal (heated, for instance, with unsweetened almond milk, hemp milk, or coconut milk, with added walnuts or blueberries), or add it to foods, such as cottage cheese, yogurt, or kefir. You can also use it as part of a breading mixture for chicken and fish (e.g., with almond flour and grated Parmesan cheese). Look for ground golden flaxseeds, rather than brown flaxseeds, as the ground golden variety has a light nutty flavor rather than the dirt-like taste of brown. Ground psyllium seed husks are also, like flaxseeds, useful for baking as they provide structure to grain-free baking. Both ground golden flaxseeds and psyllium are also useful bulking agents to firm up bowel movements, if this is an issue for you. One to 2 tablespoons per day gets the job done, but be sure to hydrate especially well, as these fibers are exceptionally hygroscopic (water absorbent). Failing to hydrate can cause a plug of stool that causes a tough case of constipation.

Kidney beans, black beans, Spanish beans, lima beans, and other starchy beans have healthy components in them, such as protein and prebiotic fiber, but the carbohydrate load can be excessive if consumed in large quantities. A 1-cup serving of beans typically contains 30 to 50 grams of carbohydrates, a quantity sufficient to substantially affect blood sugar and disable your reshaping efforts. For this reason, small servings (¼ cup) are preferable, consistent with our net carb limitation.

Vegans and vegetarians will, admittedly, have a tougher job, particularly strict vegetarians and vegans who avoid eggs, dairy, and fish. Strict vegetarians need to rely more heavily on nuts, nut meals, seeds, nut and seed butters, and oils; avocados and olives; and may have a bit more leeway with carbohydrate-containing beans, lentils, chickpeas, wild rice, chia seed, sweet potatoes, and yams. If nongenetically modified soy products can be obtained, then tofu, tempeh, and natto can provide another rich source of protein. But vegans and vegetarians will have to supplement vitamin B_{12}, zinc, and iron, and be resigned to the fact that they will be unable to ingest such nutrients as collagen and hyaluronic acid. More recently, algae sources of omega-3 fatty acids EPA and DHA have become available. (A small quantity of linolenic acid from flaxseeds, chia seeds, and other plant foods can be converted to EPA and DHA, but not enough to overcome deficiency.)

It's important to extend your food choices outside familiar habits, since variety is part of a successful diet that provides plentiful vitamins, minerals, fibers, and phytonutrients. (Conversely, part of the cause of failure of many modern commercial diets is lack of variety. The modern habit of concentrating calorie sources in one food group—wheat, for instance—means many nutrients will be lacking.)

CONSUME THESE IN UNLIMITED QUANTITIES

Vegetables (except potatoes and corn)—including mushrooms, root vegetables (radishes, onions, garlic, shallots, carrots, turnips, beets, fennel, celeriac, jicama, horseradish, ginger), lettuces, spinach, peppers, cucumbers, tomatoes, zucchini, herbs and spices (basil, oregano, rosemary, cinnamon, paprika, cilantro, thyme, chile powder)

Nuts and seeds—almonds, walnuts, pecans, hazelnuts, Brazil nuts, macadamias; peanuts (boiled or dry roasted); sunflower seeds, pumpkin seeds, sesame seeds; nut meals and flours; all-natural nut butters (without added sugar, corn syrups, or seed oils)

Oils—extra-virgin olive, avocado, coconut, butter, ghee, lard, tallow, cocoa butter, flaxseed, walnut, macadamia, sesame

Meats and eggs—preferably free-range and organic chicken, turkey, beef, pork; buffalo; ostrich; wild game; fish; shellfish; eggs (including yolks)

Cheese, butter, ghee

Nonsugary condiments—mustards, horseradish, tapenades, salsa, mayonnaise, vinegars (white, red wine, apple cider, balsamic), Worcestershire sauce, soy sauce (gluten-free, tamari, or coconut aminos), chili or pepper sauces

Olives (green, kalamata, black), pickled and fermented vegetables (e.g., asparagus, peppers, radish, tomatoes, cabbage, cucumbers)

Others: flaxseeds (ground), chia seeds, avocados, olives, coconut, unsweetened cocoa or cacao

CONSUME THESE IN LIMITED QUANTITIES

We limit these foods mostly due to excessive carb/sugar content. It therefore helps to maintain our ≤15-gram net carb rule.

Dairy (besides cheese, butter, ghee)—milk, cottage cheese, yogurt, ricotta. (This does not include our fermented yogurts or kefirs, as the lactose and other sugars are fermented out.)

Fruit—Berries are the best: blueberries, raspberries, blackberries, strawberries, cranberries. Be careful of the most sugary tropical fruits, including pineapple, papaya, mango, and banana. Minimize or avoid dried fruit, especially figs, dates, dried cranberries, dates, and raisins. With fruits such as apples, pears, citrus, cherries, and so on, adhere to our ≤15-gram net carb rule.

Fruit juices—Fruit juices are too high in sugars (e.g., 18 to 24 grams per 8 ounces) and easily exceed our 15-gram net carb limit. Fermenting juices, by the way, is a terrific way of reducing, even eliminating, carbs/sugars, allowing you to enjoy delicious effervescent juices with minimal carb/sugar exposure.

Alcoholic beverages—Go lightly here: More than one or two drinks and you stall any progress you make. Choose lower-carb, non-grain beverages, such as dry white or red wines, vodka, gin, or tequila. Some of the light beers, despite being brewed from grains, have such low protein residues that they do not appear to pose problems. If you are not exceptionally gluten sensitive, most do fine with the low-carb Michelob Light and Busch Light beers. Some local or regional brewers may also have some choices, mostly ciders; be mindful of carb content. Omission Brewing Company has an Ultimate Light brewed with malted barley with most gluten removed, though there may be risk of reaction for gluten-sensitive people.

Grain-like foods—We limit quinoa, amaranth, and buckwheat due to excessive potential carb exposure.

Legumes—black beans, white beans, kidney beans, butter beans, Spanish beans, lima beans; lentils; chickpeas and hummus

Potatoes (white and red), yams, sweet potatoes

Soy products—tofu, tempeh, miso, natto; edamame, soybeans

Higher-carb nuts—pistachios, cashews

Honey—It is easy to overdo this fructose-rich sweetener.

Ketchup, barbecue sauces and other sauces, salad dressings (avoid or minimize if contains sucrose or high-fructose corn syrup)

NEVER CONSUME

Wheat products—wheat-based breads, pasta, noodles, cookies, cakes, pies, cupcakes, breakfast cereals, pancakes, waffles, pita, couscous; bulgur, triticale, Kamut, spelt, emmer, einkorn

Wheat-related grains—corn, oats, rice, rye, barley, sorghum, millet, bulgur

Gluten-free processed foods—specifically those made with cornstarch, rice starch, potato starch, tapioca starch

Unhealthy oils—fried, hydrogenated, corn, sunflower, safflower, grapeseed, cottonseed, soybean, canola

Fried foods

Sugary snacks—candies, ice cream, sherbet, fruit roll-ups, energy bars

Sugary fructose-rich sweeteners—agave syrup or nectar, maple syrup, high-fructose corn syrup, sucrose

Sugary condiments—jellies, jams, preserves, chutney

REPLACEMENT NON-GRAIN FLOURS

When we eliminate wheat and grains, there is no need to despair that you will never have another slice of pizza, a muffin with your coffee, biscuits and gravy, or a slice of cheesecake at the holidays—you can, provided you replace unhealthy flours with healthy substitutes. This is how you make, for instance, a healthy cheesecake that does not cause weight gain, does not result in high blood sugar, does not contribute to distortions of shape. We also replace sugar and synthetic sweeteners with adverse health consequences with natural noncaloric or minimally caloric sweeteners (suggestions follow). There is almost no conventional dish that you cannot re-create that is every bit as satisfying and delicious, but not loaded down with any of the health and weight concerns of its counterparts.

Baking results are best when flours and meals are combined. A common blend, for instance, is 3 cups of almond flour + ¼ cup of ground golden flaxseeds + ¼ cup of coconut flour. Note that one challenge we face with non-grain baking is generating "rise" (increasing the volume by incorporating gas into the baking mixture). You can increase volume somewhat by whipping egg whites until frothy, using baking soda (e.g., 1 teaspoon) in combination with an acid source, such as vinegar or lemon juice, then microwaving briefly (1 to 2 minutes) before baking. For more detailed recipes, see my *Wheat Belly* cookbooks, especially the *Wheat Belly 30-Minutes (or Less!) Cookbook*.

Recall that we never resort to using gluten-free flours or baking mixes as they are exceptionally destructive for health, including introducing significant distortions in shape and body composition, such as expansion of abdominal fat. We also avoid high-carb replacement flours, such as rice flour, tapioca flour, buckwheat flour, and others.

Safe Flours and Meals

Ground almonds—Almond meal is from ground whole almonds, whereas almond flour is ground from almonds with the skin removed and oils pressed out. Use the flour when a finer texture is desired, such as a birthday cake or poppy-seed muffin; use meal when fine texture is not needed, but the health benefits of the skin and oils remain.

Ground golden flaxseeds—more useful as a "secondary" flour, one that supplements a primary flour, such as almond flour, to add cohesiveness and structure.

Coconut flour—Like ground flaxseeds, coconut flour is most useful as a secondary flour.

Ground psyllium husks—useful to increase sturdiness and structure by adding, for example, 1 tablespoon to a mixture of other flours/meals.

Ground pecans—of limited usefulness; best for making piecrusts.

Tiger nut flour—Just be careful here, as this flour, ground from a root vegetable, contains 44 grams net carbs per cup. Use this, for instance, when small portion sizes will be consumed or when preparing foods for people who are not carb conscious.

Lupin flour—Ground from a legume, this is a versatile flour that can, like almond flour, serve as a primary flour.

BEVERAGES

Water should always be your first choice. You may find that, minus the taste-distorting effects of wheat, water actually tastes better than you previously thought. Even if you did not like drinking plain water before, you may discover that your abilities to taste are renewed and the natural act of drinking plain water is quite wonderful. (Of course, filter out chlorine and fluoride before drinking.) I add some magnesium powder and a light pinch of sea salt to drinking water to sip throughout the day. Some prefer to add a squeeze of citrus, kiwi, or slice of other fruit to brighten the taste, but know that the small quantity of sugar can pose dental challenges, including shifting the composition of mouth flora.

Drinking unfermented fruit juices, fruit drinks, and certainly soft drinks, such as sodas, is a bad idea, due to excessive sugar content. We therefore ferment juices, especially with the fungus *Saccharomyces boulardii* or the bacterial species *Bacillus subtilis*, to make a sparkling soda-like drink (see recipe, page 205). Teas and coffee are fine to enjoy with or without milk, cream, or coconut milk. If an argument can be made for alcoholic beverages, the one genuine standout in health is red wine, a source of flavonoids, anthocyanins, and resveratrol. Beer, on the other hand, is a wheat- and barley-brewed beverage in most cases, and is the one clear-cut alcoholic drink to avoid or minimize. Beers also tend to be high in carbohydrates, especially the heavier ales and dark beers. If you have positive celiac markers, you should not consume any wheat- or gluten-containing beer at all.

SAFE SWEETENERS

To replace sugar (sucrose) in recipes, here is a conversion chart that lists the equivalents of safe noncaloric or minimally caloric sweeteners to 1 cup sugar. Our preferred sweetener, given its beneficial effects on blood glucose and insulin, is allulose. A growing number of excellent sweeteners combine allulose with monk fruit, an ideal combination. Erythritol is also often used for its bulk effect to combine with potent sweeteners stevia and monk fruit. Recent preliminary evidence has raised some questions about the safety of erythritol and xylitol (although questionable, given its natural occurrence in fruit such as apples and pears), while the best human clinical evidence for safety and for metabolic benefits has grown for allulose and, to a lesser degree, for monk fruit.

Although monk fruit and inulin are safe sweeteners, they are rarely, if ever, used alone. You'll therefore find them in combination products.

EQUIVALENT TO 1 CUP OF SUGAR:

Stevia, powder or liquid—variable depending on brand; consult label

Allulose—1⅓ cups

Erythritol—1⅓ cups

Xylitol—1 cup

COMBINATION SWEETENERS:

Truvia (erythritol + rebiana, an isolate of stevia): 1¼ cups

Pyure (erythritol + stevia): ½ cup

Lakanto (allulose + monk fruit): 1 cup
Health Garden (allulose + monk fruit): 1 cup

NET CARB–COUNTING RESOURCES

WEBSITES:

My Fitness Pal: https://www.myfitnesspal.com/
USDA FoodData Central: https://fdc.nal.usda.gov/index.html

SMARTPHONE APPS (FIND IN APP STORE):

My Fitness Pal
Carb Manager
Fat Secret

HANDBOOKS

The Food Counter's Pocket Companion
Dana Carpender's NEW Carb and Calorie Counter

APPENDIX B

PROBIOTIC, MACS, AND FERMENTATION RESOURCES; RECOMMENDED SOURCES OF COLLAGEN, HYALURONIC ACID, ASTAXANTHIN

SUGGESTED FERMENTING DEVICES

Ideally, the device you choose allows you to vary the duration of fermentation (aiming for a maximum of 36 hours) and the temperature to suit the needs of various species. Devices that meet these requirements include:

    Luvele yogurt maker

    Anova sous vide

    Instant Pot (versions with yogurt-making setting)

If you have a device with a nonadjustable preset temperature (including Instant Pots), verify the temperature by running the device for 30 to 60 minutes with an inexpensive thermometer inside. If the temperature is greater than 108°F, then you will need to obtain another device with adjustable temperature settings, such as from the alternative brands listed here.

RECOMMENDED PROBIOTICS

What constitutes an ideal probiotic is still a matter of debate. Most commercial preparations are little more than haphazard collections of microbes assembled with no rhyme or reason. Thankfully, even such carelessly crafted products still provide modest benefits. Remember: The best probiotics do not come in capsule form but as the fermented sauerkraut, kimchi, kefir, and other fermented foods that you include in your daily routine. But a few additional features can stack the odds in favor of obtaining favorable effects from a commercial probiotic. They include:

- A minimum of 10 billion CFUs per capsule—The evolving science suggests that higher microbial counts are more likely to generate greater beneficial effects. At what level is maximum benefit experienced? This remains unsettled. Of course, my yogurt projects yield hundreds of billions per serving, likely at least part of the reason why the benefits are greater.
- Inclusion of keystone species—This list is also a work in progress but clearly should include small intestinal–colonizing, bacteriocin-producing, body shape–molding species, such as *L. reuteri* and *L. gasseri* (unless you obtain these species from my fermented yogurts). Many other keystone species are obtainable simply by causing them to "bloom" with inclusion of dietary microbiota-accessible carbohydrates (see page 195), such species as *Faecalibacterium prausnitzii* and *Akkermansia muciniphila*, as well as enthusiastic consumption of fermented foods.
- Avoidance of gimmicks—The increasingly competitive probiotic market has caused some manufacturers to make claims that are either silly or unnecessary, such as double-encapsulation to delay release or claims that only spore-forming species survive stomach acid (which is not true—look at *L. reuteri* and *L. gasseri*, for instance, with high survivability).
- There are species/strains important for specific situations—such as *Bifidobacterium infantis* for infant neurological maturation

or *Lactobacillus crispatus* for female reproductive health. These are typically obtainable as single–species/strain products. (For a full discussion of how to restore specific species for specific benefit, see my book *Super Gut*.)

BiotiQuest Sugar Shift*

This is one of the few products in which collaborative cross-feeding effects have been incorporated into the formulation. This supplier provides a number of other interesting formulations.

BiotiQuest.com

Vital Planet Vital Flora Advanced Biome Probiotic

The 100-billion CFU counts per capsule and the inclusion of key-stone and other important species make this product a standout.

VitalpPlanet.com

Nutricost Probiotic Complex

The 50-billion CFU count and inclusion of several important species makes this a good product.

Nutricost.com

Ther-Biotic Synbiotic

The 50-billion CFU count plus inclusion of several keystone species also make this a good choice.

Klaire.com

*BiotiQuest is a sponsor of Dr. Davis's *Defiant Health* podcast.

RESOURCES FOR MICROBES AND MACS

Sources of Microbes

Recommended species and strains for your fermenting projects include:

Lactobacillus reuteri

>   Oxiceutics MyReuteri*: oxiceutics.com
>   BioGaia Osfortis: BioGaia.com

Lactobacillus gasseri

>   Mercola Market Biothin: MercolaMarket.com

Bacillus coagulans

>   Schiff Digestive Advantage: SchiffVitamins.com and widely available in most big-box stores and pharmacies

Saccharomyces boulardii

>   Florastor: widely available in most big-box stores and pharmacies

Lactobacillus rhamnosus GG

>   The widely available Culturelle product (available at Walgreens, CVS, Target, Meijer, etc.) contains this strain, as well as do many other brands, including SuperSmart, Thorne, and Pure Encapsulations.

Lactobacillus crispatus

>   Oxiceutics MyCrispatus*: oxiceutics.com Jarrow Fem-Dophilus Advanced contains this microbe. The names for Jarrow's products confusingly overlap with one another, so be sure that *L. crispatus* is listed on the label (along with several other species).

*Dr. Davis does consulting with and/or has ownership interest in providers of these products.

MAC CONTENT OF SELECTED FOODS

Recall that food should be your principal source of MACs that nourish gastrointestinal microbes that, in turn, yield factors that provide significant benefits for you. Make it a habit to include at least one food source of MACs in every meal, thereby making it easier to obtain 20 grams or more MACs per day for maximum benefit.

Acacia fiber (gum): 2 grams per teaspoon

Apple: 1 gram

Beans: 3.8 grams in ½ cup; white beans are the richest with twice this quantity (12 grams net carbs)

Chia seeds: 1.5 grams per ¼ cup

Dandelion greens: 1 gram per cup (uncooked)

Flaxseeds: 2.5 grams per ¼ cup

Green banana and plantain: 10.9 grams in one medium-size (7-inch) banana (0 grams net carbs)

Green banana flour: 2 grams per tablespoon (3 grams net carbs per tablespoon)

Inulin and/or FOS powders: 4 grams per teaspoon (0 grams net carbs)

Jerusalem artichoke: 1 gram per ½ cup, slice thinly and add to salads (12 grams net carbs per cup)

Jicama: not yet quantified

Hummus or chickpeas: 8 grams per ½ cup (13.5 grams net carbs in ½ cup)

Konjac (glucomannan): 4 grams per teaspoon

Lentils: 2.5 grams in ½ cup (11 grams net carbs)

Onions, garlic, leeks: not yet quantified

Parsnip: not yet quantified (8.5 grams net carbs per ½ cup)

Peas: 1.3 grams per ½ cup (7 grams net carbs)

Potato, raw white: 10 to 12 grams per ½ medium-size potato (0 grams net carbs) (Avoid any raw potatoes with green skin as this is a fungus. If encountered, cut off the skin.)

Psyllium seeds: not yet quantified

Turnip: not yet quantified (5.0 grams net carbs per 1 cup)

Nuts are also proving to be, in preliminary studies, a source of unique forms of prebiotic fibers and other compounds. Walnuts, almonds, pistachios, cashews, pecans, and hazelnuts are therefore sources of prebiotic fibers that, though precise quantification is lacking, add to your daily prebiotic fiber intake.

COMMERCIAL SOURCES OF MACS

In addition to inulin, acacia fiber, glucomannan, and galactooligosaccharide powders, the following are excellent commercial sources of prebiotic fibers that are obtainable through major nutrition retailers such as Vitacost and iHerb, and health-food stores:

Garden of Life Raw Organic Fiber
Swanson Ultra Inulin
NOW Inulin Prebiotic Pure Powder
Jarrow Formulas Prebiotic Inulin
Micro Ingredients Organic Inulin Powder
NOW Certified Organic Acacia Fiber
Hyperbiotics Organic Prebiotic Fiber Blend

RECOMMENDED COLLAGEN, HYALURONIC ACID, AND ASTAXANTHIN SOURCES

Collagen

With bovine, porcine, or chicken sources, we aim for an intake of 20 grams per day. (Marine-sourced collagen is equally effective at lower doses, but most retailers do not yet specify the species of fish that the product was obtained from, an issue that determines dose. Until this is clarified, a dose of at least 10 grams per day is wise.)

Vital Proteins
Great Lakes Collagen
Ancient Nutrition
Garden of Life

Hyaluronic Acid

We aim for an intake of 120 mg per day. Hyaluronic acid easily mixes into yogurt, kefirs, or other foods.

Bulk Supplements
NOW
Jarrow

Astaxanthin

We recommend 4 mg per day as the recommended dose.

NOW
Life Extension
Vitacost
Oxiceutics Gut to Glow combines *L. reuteri*, marine-sourced collagen peptides, hyaluronic acid, and astaxanthin, with recommended dosages provided with 4 capsules per day. Available from oxiceutics.com.*

*Dr. Davis has a financial interest in the company providing this product.

APPENDIX C
MICROBIOME-TESTING RESOURCES

H$_2$ AND METHANE TESTING WITH THE AIRE DEVICE

AIRE is a consumer device that allows you to "map" where bacteria are living in the GI tract—small intestine versus large intestine—to identify SIBO by assessing how long it takes for microbes to produce hydrogen (H$_2$) gas. The AIRE device also identifies excessive methane production, which suggests overgrowth of methane-producing microbes that can underlie constipation.

The quantity of the two gases measured is reported on a 1:10 scale, with each increment of 1 unit equivalent to 5 parts per million (ppm) by conventional testing performed in a clinic or lab. Any H$_2$ increase of 4 units (20 ppm) over baseline is considered positive if it occurs within 90 minutes of ingesting a fiber or sugar that bacteria metabolize for H$_2$. Any value of 2 units or greater (10 ppm) for methane is regarded as positive regardless of timing.

The device is available from the manufacturer, FoodMarble: www.foodmarble.com. Sign up for emails on its website and a discount coupon code is usually sent to you.

TESTING WITH THE AIRE DEVICE

To use the AIRE device for breath testing, follow these steps.

Day Prior

For at least 12 hours prior to breath testing, consume only foods that contain no prebiotic fibers or sugars. You should therefore avoid legumes, hummus, foods that contain inulin and acacia fiber, fruit, starchy or root vegetables, onions, garlic, sugars or fructose, and all dairy products. Also avoid any alcohol. Limit your diet to fat- and protein-rich foods, such as eggs, beef, poultry, fish, leafy greens, oils such as olive oil, and nonstarchy vegetables (e.g., spinach, kale, lettuce, green peppers, cucumbers, green beans, zucchini).

Day of Testing

1. Turn on the AIRE device.
2. Activate the AIRE/FoodMarble app on your smartphone, then follow the instructions in the app.
3. Blow into the device when prompted by the app—this is your baseline value.
4. Consume some food that contains prebiotic fiber. Our preferred fiber is inulin, such as 2 teaspoons of inulin in ¼ cup of coffee or yogurt. You can also eat other foods of your choosing that will not affect test results, such as eggs, bacon, sausage, and so forth.
5. Test every 30 to 45 minutes for up to 3 hours, and record your results. You can stop testing if a positive reading is obtained.

Interpreting the Readings

Each unit of measure on the AIRE device, from 0 to 10, corresponds to an increase in hydrogen gas of 5 parts per million (ppm) obtained by formal H_2 breath testing. A reading of 4 therefore equals 20 ppm H_2, a reading of 8 equals 40 ppm, and 10 corresponds to 50 ppm and above.

After you have consumed prebiotic fiber, interpret the readings as follows:

- A reading of 4 to 6 is suggestive of SIBO.
- A rise of 4 units above baseline identifies SIBO; for example, a baseline of 2.0 increasing to 6.0.
- Any value above 6 confidently suggests that SIBO is present.
- If there is a high baseline value, such as 8 to 10, abort the test and try again on another day after a more extended effort on the diet, for example, 24 hours preceding measurements.

The higher the value, the greater the likelihood that SIBO is present.

In the majority of people with SIBO, the results will be obvious, such as a rise from 1.2 at the start to 9.8 at the 30- or 45-minute mark.

TRIO-SMART H_2, METHANE, AND H_2S BREAST TESTING

A new service called Trio-Smart breath testing, developed in part by gastroenterologist and SIBO expert Dr. Mark Pimentel, is now available to test for hydrogen (H_2), methane, and hydrogen sulfide (H_2S). The cost for one round of testing is around $350, and many health-care insurance policies and Medicare cover most or all of the cost.

Trio-Smart breath testing: triosmartbreath.com

STOOL TESTING

A number of methods may be used to assess the composition of bowel flora. Older methods that relied on growing microbes in a petri dish have proven unreliable because many bowel species do not grow under those conditions. Instead, "culture-independent" methods have uncovered thousands of species that we weren't aware of. The following testing services rely on culture-independent assessment methods that examine microbial DNA. Stool testing can be helpful when basic efforts at restoring body composition or health yield incomplete results, and can identify microbial impediments to your success.

Unfortunately, most stool tests can only be ordered by a health-care practitioner. You should ask your doctor (who may not be familiar with them) for these tests, and they will have to register and create an account with the test company if they are not already associated with it. If your doctor refuses, find a health-care practitioner who is willing to work with you to assess this aspect of your health. Customer service representatives at each testing company can also identify practitioners in your area who use their service.

Costs are in the range of $200 to $300, except for Vibrant Wellness Gut Zoomer, the most comprehensive test, which is priced around $700, and Ombre, the least costly at around $100.

Vibrant Wellness Gut Zoomer

    www.vibrant-wellness.com

Diagnostic Solutions Laboratory GI-Map

    DiagnosticSolutionsLab.com

Ombre

    OmbreLab.com

APPENDIX D

TRACKING BODY COMPOSITION; RECOMMENDED BIOIMPEDANCE AND IR LIGHT DEVICES

TRACKING BODY COMPOSITION

Know what's better than weight loss? Regaining youthful body composition. Your goal is to not just lose fat but start by preferentially losing abdominal visceral fat while not losing muscle, perhaps even regain the muscle you've lost through the aging process. Preserving or regaining muscle provides substantial advantages in molding your body composition and maintaining control over your weight.

If you lose fat but gain muscle, just tracking body weight can be misleading. It is not uncommon, for instance, for someone to say, "I've gained eight pounds on the program—what's wrong?!" Ask that person, however, what has happened to waist circumference, and they typically respond, "Well, my waist has shrunk by five inches and I am stronger with firmer arms and shoulders." In other words, they have enjoyed important improvements in body composition not fully reflected by just tracking body weight. Likewise, if someone were tracking values obtained from a bioimpedance (body composition) device, that same person might report a reduction in total body fat, reduction in visceral fat, an increase in lean muscle mass, and an increase in basal metabolic rate, all reflecting favorable shifts in body composition—even if there is no weight loss. We are therefore going to track total body fat, visceral (abdominal) fat, waist circumference, and muscle mass. By tracking these measures and not just body weight, you can see how your body composition is improving.

I suggest you obtain the following measures at the start (day 0), then every 30 days until you achieve the shape and body composition goals you desire. Although these measures help track your progress, the ultimate determination of your success is when you look in the mirror and see firm arms, shoulders, and thighs; full facial features with minimal to no wrinkles; and a flat abdomen. When you achieve your desired shape and body appearance, take note of your measures and add them to your table so that you can continue to occasionally remeasure to make sure that you are staying on course.

	Baseline Day 0	30 Days	60 Days	90 Days	120 Days
Weight lbs					
Waist circumference inches					
Total body fat %					
Visceral fat					
Muscle mass lbs					
Body water %					

MEASURING WAIST CIRCUMFERENCE

Here is the standard method used to measure waist circumference that ensures changes are not due to breathing patterns or placement of the measuring tape, but due to real changes in abdominal fat. To measure waist circumference accurately and reproducibly:

1. Encircle your waist with the cloth measuring tape at the level of the umbilicus (belly button), making sure that it is horizontal. The tape measure should be snug against the skin but should not indent the skin.
2. Take a deep breath, breathe out, repeat the deep breath, then breathe out again and measure at the end of exhalation.
3. Record the value in your log.

Compared to methods such as dual X-ray absorptiometry (DEXA), devices that use bioimpedance yield less-than-perfect accuracy, but these devices can be useful to accurately track changes over time.

WHAT IS IDEAL BODY COMPOSITION?

It is difficult to specify measures that are ideal as there is such wide variation in human body shapes, height, genetics, age, ethnicity, race, and other factors. However, we can generate some rough guidelines to compare you to other people. Also, recognize that bioimpedance devices are most helpful in tracking changes in such measures as visceral fat and lean muscle mass but less helpful in generating absolute or precise values. The goal is therefore not so much as attaining a specific quantity of lean muscle mass but to track these measures, then look in the mirror to assess whether you are satisfied with your body composition: Is your abdomen flat with at least some abdominal muscles evident, or is there a persistent ring of loose skin and fat encircling your waist (a.k.a. love handles)? Are your shoulders, arms, thighs, and calves muscular?

If you are interested in correlating body composition with metabolic health, the most valuable measure to track along with body composition measures is the level of triglycerides in your blood-stream, a common value that is part of any standard four-component cholesterol panel (along with HDL cholesterol, LDL cholesterol, and total cholesterol). A useful rule of thumb: A fasting triglyceride level of 60 mg/dl or less correlates with favorable body composition and metabolic health. Other measures can also be tracked along with body composition measures, to gauge whether improvements in body composition—reduction in total body fat, reduction in visceral fat, increased lean muscle mass, reduction in waist circumference—are reflected in such measures as fasting glucose, fasting insulin, hemo-globin A1c, blood pressure, and C-reactive protein. In other words, if you lose, say, 8 pounds of total body fat and your fasting glucose drops from 110 mg/dl to 100 mg/dl, you will know that you are achieving improvements not only in body composition but also in important markers of metabolic health.

MEASURING BODY COMPOSITION WITH BIOIMPEDANCE SCALES

These consumer devices take advantage of the variable abilities of dif-ferent tissues in the body to conduct a weak electrical current. Fat, for instance, is a poor conductor, whereas muscle is a better conductor. This principle allows us to decipher measures of total body fat, lean muscle mass, and total body water, with some devices also measuring visceral fat and basal metabolic rate. Compared to such methods as DEXA, bioimpedance measurements correlate fairly well. However, measurements can be influenced by a number of factors that introduce excessive variation.

To minimize random variation in your measurements:

1. Consume no food for the preceding 2 hours. However, remain hydrated. Even better, drink a standard amount of water prior to making measurements, such as two 8-ounce glasses in the hour preceding.

2. For repeated measurements, choose about the same time of day for each measure, such as eight a.m. If possible, also make your measurements at similar room temperatures.
3. If you are a female with active menstrual cycles, choose a similar day in your cycle to make measurements, such as a week after the start of bleeding.
4. Avoid creams or other products on the skin contacting the device.
5. Record your values: baseline, 30 days, 60 days, 90 days, etc.

These factors may seem trivial or inconsequential, but for bioimpedance body composition measurements, they can play large roles. So it is indeed helpful to pay attention to the previous factors.

RECOMMENDED BIOIMPEDANCE (BODY COMPOSITION) SCALES

These are scales that send a small (painless) electrical current from your feet through the rest of your body, then calculate such measures as muscle mass, total fat, and visceral fat, based on the varying relative resistances to conducting current through different tissues. Tracking these measures can be helpful as you lose total fat, abdominal visceral fat, and maintain or regain muscle, since weight alone likely does not reflect the full range of body composition changes. Remember: An increase in muscle coupled with loss of visceral fat is the ideal outcome.

Note that there are many devices available. The following were chosen for the ability to quantify visceral fat specifically. Note that these products, as well as others not listed, differ in their upper weight limits, how many users are accepted, power source (e.g., batteries vs. a rechargeable USB-connected battery), whether Bluetooth-enabled to communicate with your smartphone or not, and syncing with other devices. For the sake of affordability, I chose devices that do not use multiple electrodes or multiple electrical frequencies (as employed in more costly medical-grade devices). Another option, of course, is to rely on the device that may be present in some doctors' offices.

Note that bioimpedance devices should not be used if you have a pacemaker.

Tanita

RD-901 InnerScan PRO Smart Body Composition Scale—higher priced at around $200

GE

GE Fit Plus LN—around $53

GE Fit Plus KN—similar to the LN but syncs with Fitbit, Google Fit, and Apple Health; around $60

Omron

BCM-500 Body Composition Monitor and Scale with Bluetooth Connectivity—about $65

Withings

Body Smart—around $90

INFRARED LIGHT DEVICES

The area of photobiomodulation (the effects of light on biological functions) is in its infancy. But evolving science has indeed confirmed that harmful effects can develop when we are deprived of light in the red and infrared (IR) wavelengths and that beneficial effects develop when these wavelengths are restored. The popular conversion of incandescent lights over to LEDs to save energy has markedly reduced our exposure to red and IR wavelengths since incandescent emits red and IR but current LEDs do not. Preliminary evidence suggests that this practice that overexposes us to blue wavelengths of light may be a factor in causing weight gain as fat.

The best source of red and IR wavelengths is exposure to sunlight. Make it a point to obtain several minutes of exposure to sunlight every day whenever possible. Red and IR wavelengths penetrate clothes, so there is no need to reduce clothing coverage. Because we spend so much time indoors, consider replacing at least a few of your LED lights with old-fashioned incandescent lights, especially at locations you frequent. For me, for instance, I replaced the bulbs at my work desk with incandescent (and experienced improvement in my vision within 48 hours).

You can also use red/IR devices. Unfortunately, there are a lot of unscrupulous or low-quality manufacturers and retailers who fail to inform you that devices costing thousands of dollars are likely no better than devices that cost less than $100. The site of exposure may also not be important as red/IR applied to any area of the body may signal the improvements in metabolism that result from the activation of energy production that develops with just 3 minutes per day of exposure. (Eye and brain benefits, however, may require direct exposure.)

Vevor

This simple, no-frills device provides the two most important red/IR wavelengths of 660 and 850 nm and costs less than $100.

vevor.com

Astarexin

Like the Vevor device, this provides red/IR at 660 and 850 nm wavelengths, also with a cost of around $100.

NOTES

CHAPTER 1

1. Iscan MY, Kennedy KAR, eds. *Reconstruction of Life from the Human Skeleton.* Wiley-Liss; 1989.

2. Nagar Y, Hershkovitz I. Interrelationship between various aging methods, and their relevance to paleodemography. *Human Evol.* 2004;19:145-56.

3. Neeland IJ, Ross R, Després JP, et al.; International Atherosclerosis Society; International Chair on Cardiometabolic Risk Working Group on Visceral Obesity. Visceral and ectopic fat, atherosclerosis, and cardiometabolic disease: A position statement. *Lancet Diabetes Endocrinol.* 2019 Sep;7(9):715-25.

4. de Mutsert R, Gast K, Widya R, et al. Associations of abdominal subcutaneous and visceral fat with insulin resistance and secretion differ between men and women: The Netherlands Epidemiology of Obesity Study. *Metab Syndr Relat Disord.* 2018 Feb;16(1):54-63.

5. Smith U. Abdominal obesity: A marker of ectopic fat accumulation. *J Clin Invest.* 2015 May;125(5):1790-2.

6. Merlotti C, Ceriani V, Morabito A, Pontiroli AE. Subcutaneous fat loss is greater than visceral fat loss with diet and exercise, weight-loss promoting drugs and bariatric surgery: A critical review and meta-analysis. *Int J Obes (Lond).* 2017 May;41(5):672-82.

7. Willoughby D, Hewlings S, Kalman D. Body composition changes in weight loss: Strategies and supplementation for maintaining lean body mass, a brief review. *Nutrients.* 2018 Dec 3;10(12):1876.

8. Wilding JPH, Batterham RL, Davies M, et al.; STEP 1 Study Group. Weight regain and cardiometabolic effects after withdrawal of semaglutide: The STEP 1 trial extension. *Diabetes Obes Metab.* 2022 Aug;24(8):1553-64.

9.   Chen C, Ye Y, Zhang Y, Pan XF, Pan A. Weight change across adulthood in relation to all cause and cause specific mortality: Prospective cohort study. *BMJ.* 2019 Oct 16;367:l5584.

10.   Hampl SE, Hassink SG, Skinner AC, et al. Clinical practice guideline for the evaluation and treatment of children and adolescents with obesity. *Pediatrics.* 2023 Feb;151(2):e2022060640.

11.   Kitaghenda FK, Hong J, Shao Y, Yao L, Zhu X. The prevalence of small intestinal bacterial overgrowth after roux-en-Y gastric bypass (RYGB): A systematic review and meta-analysis. *Obes Surg.* 2024 Jan;34(1):250-7.

12.   Huppler L, Robertson AG, Wiggins T, Hollyman M, Welbourn R. How safe bariatric surgery is: An update on perioperative mortality for clinicians and patients. *Clin Obes.* 2022 Jun;12(3):e12515.

13.   Estimate of Bariatric Surgery Numbers, 2011-2021. American Society for Metabolic and Bariatric Surgery, 2023: https://asmbs.org/resources/estimate-of-bariatric-surgery-numbers.

14.   Higa K, Ho T, Tercero F, Yunus T, Boone KB. Laparoscopic Roux-en-Y gastric bypass: 10-year follow-up. *Surg Obes Relat Dis.* 2011 Jul-Aug;7(4):516-25.

15.   Peterhänsel C, Petroff D, Klinitzke G, Kersting A, Wagner B. Risk of completed suicide after bariatric surgery: A systematic review. *Obes Rev.* 2013 May;14(5):369-82.

16.   CBS News. Bypass surgery gone bad, 2005: https://www.cbsnews.com/news/gastric-bypass-surgery-gone-bad.

17.   Nagem RG, Lázaro-da-Silva A, de Oliveira RM, Morato VG. Gallstone-related complications after Roux-en-Y gastric bypass: A prospective study. *Hepatobiliary Pancreat Dis Int.* 2012 Dec 15;11(6):630-5.

18.   ABC News. Choking death linked to gastric bypass surgery, 2012: https://abcnews.go.com/Health/Wellness/uk-woman-chokes-death-weight-loss-surgery/story?id=16566239.

19.   Castaneda D, Popov VB, Wander P, Thompson CC. Risk of suicide and self-harm is increased after bariatric surgery: A systematic review and meta-analysis. *Obes Surg.* 2019 Jan;29(1):322-33.

20.   Kefurt R, Langer FB, Schindler K, Shakeri-Leidenmühler S, Ludvik B, Prager G. Hypoglycemia after roux-en-Y gastric bypass: Detection rates of continuous glucose monitoring (CGM) versus mixed meal test. *Surg Obes Relat Dis.* 2015 May-Jun;11(3):564-9.

21.   Berger JR. The neurological complications of bariatric surgery. *Arch Neurol.* 2004;61(8):1185-9.

22.   Vannevel V, Jans G, Bialecka M, Lannoo M, Devlieger R, Van Mieghem T. Internal herniation in pregnancy after gastric bypass: A systematic review. *Obstet Gynecol.* 2016 Jun;127(6):1013-20.

23. Diamond DM, Ravnskov U. How statistical deception created the appearance that statins are safe and effective in primary and secondary prevention of cardiovascular disease. *Expert Rev Clin Pharmacol.* 2015;8(2):201.

CHAPTER 2

1. Oteng AB, Kersten S. Mechanisms of action of trans fatty acids. *Adv Nutr.* 2020 May 1;11(3):697-708.

2. A final farewell to artificial trans fat. Center for Science in the Public Interest, 2018 June 13: https://www.cspinet.org/news/final-farewell -artificial-trans-fat-20180613.

3. Know your facts about diabetes. American Diabetes Association: https://diabetes.org/about-diabetes/diabetes-myths. Accessed Jan 8, 2024.

4. Russell-Jones D, Khan R. Insulin-associated weight gain in diabetes—causes, effects and coping strategies. *Diabetes Obes Metab.* 2007 Nov;9(6):799-812.

5. Caporaso NE, Jones RR, Stolzenberg-Solomon RZ, Medgyesi DN, Kahle LL, Graubard BI. Insulin resistance in healthy U.S. adults: Findings from the National Health and Nutrition Examination Survey (NHANES). *Cancer Epidemiol Biomarkers Prev.* 2020 Jan;29(1):157-68.

6. da Silva AA, do Carmo JM, Li X, Wang Z, Mouton AJ, Hall JE. Role of hyperinsulinemia and insulin resistance in hypertension: Metabolic syndrome revisited. *Can J Cardiol.* 2020 May;36(5):671-82.

7. Chen J, Liang H, Tan Y, et al. Association of urinary iodine concentration with prediabetes/diabetes in adults: Analysis of the NHANES 2005-2016. *J Trace Elem Med Biol.* 2023 May;77:127144.

8. Freeland-Graves JH, Nitzke S; Academy of Nutrition and Dietetics. Position of the academy of nutrition and dietetics: Total diet approach to healthy eating. *J Acad Nutr Diet.* 2013 Feb;113(2):307-17.

9. Chassaing B, Koren O, Goodrich JK, et al. Dietary emulsifiers impact the mouse gut microbiota promoting colitis and metabolic syndrome. *Nature.* 2015 Mar 5;519(7541):92-6.

10. Naimi S, Viennois E, Gewirtz AT, Chassaing B. Direct impact of commonly used dietary emulsifiers on human gut microbiota. *Microbiome.* 2021 Mar 22;9(1):66.

11. Poti JM, Braga B, Qin B. Ultra-processed food intake and obesity: What really matters for health—processing or nutrient content? *Curr Obes Rep.* 2017 Dec;6(4):420-31.

12. Costa CS, Rauber F, Leffa PS, Sangalli CN, Campagnolo PDB, Vitolo MR. Ultra-processed food consumption and its effects on anthropometric and glucose profile: A longitudinal study during childhood. *Nutr Metab Cardiovasc Dis.* 2019 Feb;29(2):177-84.

13. Kullgren J, Solway E, Roberts S, et al. National poll on healthy aging: Addiction to highly processed food among older adults. 2023: https://deepblue.lib.umich.edu/bitstream/handle/2027.42/175578/0298_NPHA-Addictive-Eating-report-FINAL-doi.pdf?sequence=4&isAllowed=y.

14. Falkenhain K, Roach LA, McCreary S, et al. Effect of carbohydrate-restricted dietary interventions on LDL particle size and number in adults in the context of weight loss or weight maintenance: A systematic review and meta-analysis. *Am J Clin Nutr.* 2021 Oct 4;114(4):1455-66.

15. Heijnen ML, van Amelsvoort JM, Weststrate JA. Interaction between physical structure and amylose: Amylopectin ratio of foods on postprandial glucose and insulin responses in healthy subjects. *Eur J Clin Nutr.* 1995 Jun;49(6):446-57.

16. Huebner FR, Lieberman KW, Rubino RP, Wall JS. Demonstration of high opioid-like activity in isolated peptides from wheat gluten hydrolysates. *Peptides.* 1984 Nov-Dec;5(6):1139-47.

17. Hsu DJ, Lee CW, Tsai WC, Chien YC. Essential and toxic metals in animal bone broths. *Food Nutr Res.* 2017 Jul 18;61(1):1347478.

18. Monro JA, Leon R, Puri BK. The risk of lead contamination in bone broth diets. *Med Hypotheses.* 2013 Apr;80(4):389-90.

19. Hosseini F, Jayedi A, Khan T, et al. Dietary carbohydrate and the risk of type 2 diabetes: An updated systematic review and dose-response meta-analysis of prospective cohort studies. *Sci Rep.* 2022;12:2491.

20. Ahn H, Kim DW, Ko Y, et al. Updated systematic review and meta-analysis on diagnostic issues and the prognostic impact of myosteatosis: A new paradigm beyond sarcopenia. *Ageing Res Rev.* 2021 Sep;70:101398.

21. Ambati RR, Phang SM, Ravi S, Aswathanarayana RG. Astaxanthin: Sources, extraction, stability, biological activities and its commercial applications—a review. *Mar Drugs.* 2014 Jan 7;12(1):128-52.

22. Nebeling LC, Forman MR, Graubard BI, Snyder RA. Changes in carotenoid intake in the United States: The 1987 and 1992 National Health Interview Surveys. J Am Diet Assoc. 1997 Sep;97(9):991-6; Bonet ML, Canas JA, Ribot J, Palou A. Carotenoids in adipose tissue biology and obesity. *Subcell Biochem.* 2016;79:377-414.

23. Nakanishi R, Kanazashi M, Tanaka M, et al. Impacts of astaxanthin supplementation on walking capacity by reducing oxidative stress in nursing home residents. *Environ Res Pub Health.* 2022;19:13492.

24. Moran NE, Mohn ES, Hason N, Erdman JW Jr, Johnson EJ. Intrinsic and extrinsic factors impacting absorption, metabolism, and health effects of dietary carotenoids. *Adv Nutr.* 2018 Jul 1;9(4):465-92.

25. Bonet ML, Canas JA, Ribot J, Palou A. Carotenoids in adipose tissue biology and obesity. *Subcell Biochem.* 2016;79:377-414.

CHAPTER 3

1. Mehta T, Smith DL Jr, Muhammad J, Casazza K. Impact of weight cycling on risk of morbidity and mortality. *Obes Rev.* 2014 Nov;15(11):870-81.

2. Zarzo I, Boselli PM, Soriano JM. History of slimming diets up to the late 1950s. *Obesities.* 2022;2(2):115-26.

3. Vogel L. Fat shaming is making people sicker and heavier. *CMAJ.* 2019 Jun 10;191(23):E649.

4. QuickStats: Age-adjusted percentage of adults aged ≥20 years who tried to lose weight during the past 12 months, by sex—National Health and Nutrition Examination Survey, 2007–2008 to 2015–2016.

5. Cava E, Yeat NC, Mittendorfer B. Preserving healthy muscle during weight loss. *Adv Nutr.* 2017 May 15;8(3):511-19.

6. Sayer AA, Cruz-Jentoft A. Sarcopenia definition, diagnosis and treatment: Consensus is growing. *Age Ageing.* 2022 Oct 6;51(10):afac220.

7. Cereda E, Malavazos AE, Caccialanza R, et al. Cycling is associated with body weight excess and abdominal fat accumulation: A cross-sectional study. *Clin Nutr.* 2011 Dec;30(6):718-23.

8. Fothergill E, Guo J, Howard L, et al. Persistent metabolic adaptation 6 years after "The Biggest Loser" competition. *Obesity (Silver Spring).* 2016 Aug;24(8):1612-9.

9. Chaissang B, Koren O, Goodrich JK, et al. Dietary emulsifiers impact the mouse gut microbiota promoting colitis and metabolic syndrome. *Nature.* 2015;519(7541):92-6.

10. Sumithran P, Prendergast LA, Delbridge E, et al. Long-term persistence of hormonal adaptations to weight loss. *N Engl J Med.* 2011; 365:1597-604.

11. Cummings DE, Weigle DS, Frayo RS, et al. Plasma ghrelin levels after diet-induced weight loss or gastric bypass surgery. *N Engl J Med.* 2002 May 23;346(21):1623-30.

12. Landry MJ, Crimarco A, Gardner CD. Benefits of low carbohydrate diets: A settled question or still controversial? *Curr Obes Rep.* 2021 Sep;10(3):409-22.

CHAPTER 4

1.   Wilkinson DJ, Piasecki M, Atherton PJ. The age-related loss of skeletal muscle mass and function: Measurement and physiology of muscle fibre atrophy and muscle fibre loss in humans. *Ageing Res Rev*. 2018 Nov;47:123-32.

2.   Xu J, Wan CS, Ktoris K, et al. Sarcopenia is associated with mortality in adults: A systematic review and meta-analysis. *Gerontology*. 2022 May 2;68(4):361-76.

3.   Fothergill E, Guo J, Howard L, et al. Persistent metabolic adaptation 6 years after "The Biggest Loser" competition. *Obesity (Silver Spring)*. 2016 Aug;24(8):1612-9.

4.   Johannsen DL, Knuth ND, Huizenga R, Rood JC, Ravussin E, Hall KD. Metabolic slowing with massive weight loss despite preservation of fat-free mass. *J Clin Endocrinol Metab*. 2012 Jul;97(7):2489-96.

5.   Erdman SE, Poutahidis T. Probiotic "glow of health": It's more than skin deep. *Benef Microbes*. 2014 Jun 1;5(2):109-19.

6.   Varian BJ, Goureshetti S, Poutahidis T, et al. Beneficial bacteria inhibit cachexia. *Oncotarget*. 2016 Mar 15;7(11):11803-16.

7.   Elabd C, Cousin W, Upadhyayula P, et al. Oxytocin is an age-specific circulating hormone that is necessary for muscle maintenance and regeneration. *Nat Commun*. 2014 Jun 10;5:4082.

8.   Varian BJ, Poutahidis T, DiBenedictis BT, et al. Microbial lysate upregulates host oxytocin. *Brain Behav Immun*. 2017 Mar;61:36-49.

9.   Ferolla SM, Couto CA, Costa-Silva L, et al. Beneficial effect of synbiotic supplementation on hepatic steatosis and anthropometric parameters, but not on gut permeability in a population with nonalcoholic steatohepatitis. *Nutrients*. 2016 Jun 28;8(7).

10.   de Jong TR, Neumann ID. Oxytocin and aggression. *Curr Top Behav Neurosci*. 2018;35:175-92.

11.   Jones C, Barrera I, Brothers S, Ring R, Wahlestedt C. Oxytocin and social functioning. *Dialogues Clin Neurosci*. 2017 Jun;19(2):193-201.

12.   Molin G, Jeppsson B, Johansson M, et al. Numerical taxonomy of Lactobacillus spp. associated with healthy and diseased mucosa of the human intestines. *J Appl Bacteriol*. 1993;74:314-23.

13.   Walter J, Britton RA, Roos S. Host-microbial symbiosis in the vertebrate gastrointestinal tract and the *Lactobacillus reuteri* paradigm. *Proc Natl Acad Sci*. 2011;108:4645-52.

14.   Dommels Y, Kemperman R, Zebregs Y, et al. Survival of *Lactobacillus reuteri* DSM 17938 and *Lactobacillus rhamnosus* GG in the human gastrointestinal tract with daily consumption of a low-fat probiotic spread. *Appl Environ Microbiol*. 2009;75:6198-204.

15. Valk R, Hammill J, Grip J. Saturated fat: Villain and bogeyman in the development of cardiovascular disease? *Eur J Prev Cardiol*. 2022 Dec 21;29(18):2312-21.

16. Zdzieblik D, Oesser S, Baumstark MW, Gollhofer A, König D. Collagen peptide supplementation in combination with resistance training improves body composition and increases muscle strength in elderly sarcopenic men: A randomised controlled trial. *Br J Nutr*. 2015 Oct 28;114(8): 1237-45.

17. Jendricke P, Centner C, Zdzieblik D, Gollhofer A, König D. Specific collagen peptides in combination with resistance training improve body composition and regional muscle strength in premenopausal women: A randomized controlled trial. *Nutrients*. 2019 Apr 20;11(4):892.

18. Zhu C, Li G, Peng H, Zang F, Chen Y, Li Y. Treatment with marine collagen peptides modulates glucose and lipid metabolism in Chinese patients with type 2 diabetes mellitus. *Appl Physiol Nutr Metab*. 2010;35(6):797-804.

19. Pan L, Ai X, Fu T, et al. In vitro fermentation of hyaluronan by human gut microbiota: Changes in microbiota community and potential degradation mechanism. *Carbohydr Polym*. 2021 Oct 1;269:118313.

20. Böhm V, Lietz G, Olmedilla-Alonso B, et al. From carotenoid intake to carotenoid blood and tissue concentrations—implications for dietary intake recommendations. *Nutr Rev*. 2021 Apr 7;79(5):544-73.

21. Chang MX, Xiong F. Astaxanthin and its effects in inflammatory responses and inflammation-associated diseases: Recent advances and future directions. *Molecules*. 2020 Nov 16;25(22):5342.

22. Nakanishi R, Kanazashi M, Tanaka M, et al. Impacts of astaxanthin supplementation on walking capacity by reducing oxidative stress in nursing home residents. *Environ Res Pub Health*. 2022;19:13492.

CHAPTER 5

1. Molin G, Jeppsson B, Johansson M, et al. Numerical taxonomy of Lactobacillus spp. associated with healthy and diseased mucosa of the human intestines. *J Appl Bacteriol*. 1993;74:314-23.

2. Walter J, Britton RA, Roos S. Host-microbial symbiosis in the vertebrate gastrointestinal tract and the *Lactobacillus reuteri* paradigm. *Proc Natl Acad Sci*. 2011;108:4645-52.

3. Dommels Y, Kemperman R, Zebregs Y, et al. Survival of *Lactobacillus reuteri* DSM 17938 and *Lactobacillus rhamnosus* GG in the human gastrointestinal tract with daily consumption of a low-fat probiotic spread. *Appl Environ Microbiol*. 2009;75:6198-204.

4. Hicks LA, Taylor TH, Hunkler RJ. U.S. outpatient antibiotic prescribing, 2010. *N Engl J Med.* 2013;368:1461-62.

5. Fragiadakis GK, Smits SA, Sonnenburg ED, et al. Links between environment, diet, and the hunter-gatherer microbiome. *Gut Microbes.* 2019;10(2):216-27.

6. Conteville LC, Oliveira-Ferreira J, Vicente ACP. Gut microbiome biomarkers and functional diversity within an Amazonian semi-nomadic hunter-gatherer group. *Front Microbiol.* 2019 Jul 30;10:1743.

7. Varian BJ, Goureshetti S, Poutahidis T, et al. Beneficial bacteria inhibit cachexia. *Oncotarget.* 2016 Mar 15;7(11):11803-16.

8. Elabd C, Cousin W, Upadhyayula P, et al. Oxytocin is an age-specific circulating hormone that is necessary for muscle maintenance and regeneration. *Nat Commun.* 2014 Jun 10;5:4082.

9. Hsieh FC, Lee CL, Chai CY, et al. Oral administration of *Lactobacillus reuteri* GMNL-263 improves insulin resistance and ameliorates hepatic steatosis in high fructose-fed rats. *Nutr Metab.* 2013;10:35.

10. Poutahidis T, Springer A, Levkovich T, et al. Probiotic microbes sustain youthful serum testosterone levels and testicular size in aging mice. *PLoS One.* 2014 Jan 2;9(1):e84877.

11. Kerem L, Lawson EA. Oxytocin, eating behavior, and metabolism in humans. *Handb Clin Neurol.* 2021;180:89-103.

12. Erdman SE, Poutahidis T. Probiotic "glow of health": It's more than skin deep. *Benef Microbes.* 2014 Jun 1;5(2):109-19.

13. Peng Y, Ma Y, Luo Z, Jiang Y, Xu Z, Yu R. *Lactobacillus reuteri* in digestive system diseases: Focus on clinical trials and mechanisms. *Front Cell Infect Microbiol.* 2023 Aug 18;13:1254198.

14. Klare I, Konstabel C, Werner G, et al. Antimicrobial susceptibilities of *Lactobacillus*, *Pediococcus* and *Lactococcus* human isolates and cultures intended for probiotic or nutritional use. *J Antimicrob Chemother.* 2007 May;59(5):900-12.

15. Sroka N, Rydzewska-Rosołowska A, Kakareko K, Rosołowski M, Głowińska I, Hryszko T. Show me what you have inside—the complex interplay between SIBO and multiple medical conditions: A systematic review. *Nutrients.* 2022 Dec 24;15(1):90.

16. Violi F, Cammisotto V, Bartimoccia S, Pignatelli P, Carnevale R, Nocella C. Gut-derived low-grade endotoxaemia, atherothrombosis and cardiovascular disease. *Nat Rev Cardiol.* 2023 Jan;20(1):24-37.

17. Mathur R, Amichai M, Chua KS, Mirocha J, Barlow GM, Pimentel M. Methane and hydrogen positivity on breath test is associated with

greater body mass index and body fat. *J Clin Endocrinol Metab*. 2013 Apr;98(4): E698-702.

18. Roland BC, Lee D, Miller LS, et al. Obesity increases the risk of small intestinal bacterial overgrowth (SIBO). *Neurogastroenterol Motil*. 2018 Mar; 30(3).

19. Feng X, Li XQ. The prevalence of small intestinal bacterial overgrowth in diabetes mellitus: A systematic review and meta-analysis. *Aging (Albany NY)*. 2022 Jan 27;14(2):975-88.

20. Gudan A, Jamioł-Milc D, Hawryłkowicz V, Skonieczna-Żydecka K, Stachowska E. The prevalence of small intestinal bacterial overgrowth in patients with non-alcoholic liver diseases: NAFLD, NASH, Fibrosis, Cirrhosis- A systematic review, meta-analysis and meta-regression. *Nutrients*. 2022 Dec 9;14(24):5261.

21. Shah A, Talley NJ, Jones M, et al. Small intestinal bacterial overgrowth in irritable bowel syndrome: A systematic review and meta-analysis of case-control studies. *Am J Gastroenterol*. 2020 Feb;115(2):190-201.

22. Pimentel M, Wallace D, Hallegua D, et al. A link between irritable bowel syndrome and fibromyalgia may be related to findings on lactulose breath testing. *Ann Rheum Dis*. 2004 Apr;63(4):450-2.

23. Li X, Feng X, Jiang Z, Jiang Z. Association of small intestinal bacterial overgrowth with Parkinson's disease: A systematic review and meta-analysis. *Gut Pathog*. 2021 Apr 16;13(1):25.

24. Kowalski K, Mulak A. Small intestinal bacterial overgrowth in Alzheimer's disease. *J Neural Transm*. (Vienna). 2022 Jan;129(1):75-83.

25. Weinstock LB, Walters AS. Restless legs syndrome is associated with irritable bowel syndrome and small intestinal bacterial overgrowth. *Sleep Med*. 2011 Jun;12(6):610-3.

26. Kim DB, Park CS, Paik CN, Kang YJ, Jo IH, Lee JM. Relationship between untreated obstructive sleep apnea and breath hydrogen and methane after glucose load. *Saudi J Gastroenterol*. 2022 Sep-Oct;28(5):355-61.

27. Zhao J, Huang Y, Yu X. A narrative review of gut-muscle axis and sarcopenia: The potential role of gut microbiota. *Intl J Gen Med*. 2022: 1263-73.

28. Wall R, Fitzgerald G, Hussey S, et al. Genomic diversity of cultivable *Lactobacillus* populations residing in the neonatal and adult gastrointestinal tract. *FEMS Microbiol Ecol*. 2007 Jan;59(1):127-37.

29. Selle K, Klaenhammer TR. Genomic and phenotypic evidence for probiotic influences of *Lactobacillus gasseri* on human health. *FEMS Microbiol Rev*. 2013 Nov;37(6):915-35.

30. Kim J, Yun JM, Kim MK, Kwon O, Cho B. *Lactobacillus gasseri* BNR17 supplementation reduces the visceral fat accumulation and waist circumference in obese adults: A randomized, double-blind, placebo-controlled trial. *J Med Food.* 2018 May;21(5):454-61.

31. Nishida K, Sawada D, Kuwano Y, et al. Daily administration of paraprobiotic *Lactobacillus gasseri* CP2305 ameliorates chronic stress-associated symptoms in Japanese medical students. *J Funct Foods.* 2017;36:112-21.

32. Le Marrec C, Hyronimus B, Bressollier P, Verneuil B, Urdaci MC. Biochemical and genetic characterization of coagulin, a new antilisterial bacteriocin in the pediocin family of bacteriocins, produced by *Bacillus coagulans* I(4). *Appl Environ Microbiol.* 2000 Dec;66(12):5213-20.

33. Gupta AK, Maity C. Efficacy and safety of Bacillus coagulans LBSC in irritable bowel syndrome: A prospective, interventional, randomized, double-blind, placebo-controlled clinical study [CONSORT Compliant]. *Medicine (Baltimore).* 2021 Jan 22;100(3):e23641.

34. Cano R. Unpublished data.

35. Tarik M, Ramakrishnan L, Bhatia N, et al. The effect of *Bacillus coagulans* Unique IS-2 supplementation on plasma amino acid levels and muscle strength in resistance trained males consuming whey protein: A double-blind, placebo-controlled study. *Eur J Nutr.* 2022 Aug;61(5):2673-85.

36. Jäger R, Shields KA, Lowery RP, et al. Probiotic *Bacillus coagulans* GBI-30, 6086 reduces exercise-induced muscle damage and increases recovery. *Peer J.* 2016 Jul 21;4:e2276.

37. Borghini R, Donato G, Alvaro D, Picarrelli A. New insights in IBS-like disorders: Pandora's box has been opened; a review. *Gastroenterol Hepatol Bed Bench Spring.* 2017;10(2):79-89.

38. Rezaie A, Buresi M, Lembo A, et al. Hydrogen and methane-based breath testing in gastrointestinal disorders: The North American consensus. *Am J Gastroenterol.* 2017;112(5):775-84.

39. Schink M, Konturek PC, Tietz E, et al. Microbial patterns in patients with histamine intolerance. *J Physiol Pharmacol.* 2018;69(4).

40. Ghoshal UC, Shukla R, Ghoshal U. Small intestinal bacterial overgrowth and irritable bowel syndrome: A bridge between functional organic dichotomy. *Gut Liver.* 2017;11(2):196-208.

41. Husebye E, Skar V, Hoverstad T, et al. Fasting hypochlorhydria with gram positive gastric flora is highly prevalent in healthy old people. *Gut.* 1992;33:1331-7.

42. Rao SSC, Bhagatwala J. Small intestinal bacterial overgrowth: Clinical features and therapeutic management. *Clin Transl Gastroenterol.* 2019 Oct;10(10):e00078.

43. Muraki M, Fujiwara Y, Machida H, et al. Role of small intestinal bacterial overgrowth in severe small intestinal damage in chronic non-steroidal anti-inflammatory drug users. *Scand J Gastroenterol.* 2014;49(3):267-73.

44. Lauritano EC, Bilotta AL, Gabrielli M, et al. Association between hypothyroidism and small intestinal bacterial overgrowth. *J Clin Endocrinol Metab.* 2007;92:4180-84.

45. Brechmann T, Sperlbaum A, Schmiegel W. Levothyroxine therapy and impaired clearance are the strongest contributors to small intestinal bacterial overgrowth: Results of a retrospective cohort study. *World J Gastroenterol.* 2017;3(5):842-52.

46. Roland BC, Lee D, Miller LS, et al. Obesity increases the risk of small intestinal bacterial overgrowth (SIBO). *Neurogastroenterol Motil.* 2018; 30(3).

47. Chakaroun RM, Massier L, Kovacs P. Gut microbiome, intestinal permeability, and tissue bacteria in metabolic disease: Perpetrators or bystanders? *Nutrients.* 2020;12(4):1082.

48. Shah A, Morrison M, Burger D, et al. Systematic review with meta-analysis: The prevalence of small intestinal bacterial overgrowth in inflammatory bowel disease. *Aliment Pharmacol Ther.* 2019;49:624-35.

49. Losurdo G, D'Abramo FS, Indellicati G, et al. The influence of small intestinal bacterial overgrowth in digestive and extra-intestinal disorders. *Int J Mol Sci.* 2020;21(10):3531.

50. Fu P, Gao M, Yung KKL. Association of intestinal disorders with Parkinson's disease and Alzheimer's disease: A systematic review and meta-analysis. *ACS Chem Neurosci.* 2020;11(3):395-405.

51. Blum DJ, During E, Barwick F, et al. Restless leg syndrome: Does it start with a gut feeling? *Sleep.* 2019;42(1):A4.

CHAPTER 6

1. Yan SF, D'Agati V, Schmidt AM, Ramasamy R. Receptor for Advanced Glycation Endproducts (RAGE): A formidable force in the pathogenesis of the cardiovascular complications of diabetes & aging. *Curr Mol Med.* 2007 Dec;7(8):699-710.

2. Zdzieblik D, Oesser S, Baumstark MW, Gollhofer A, König D. Collagen peptide supplementation in combination with resistance training improves body composition and increases muscle strength in elderly sarcopenic men: A randomised controlled trial. *Br J Nutr.* 2015 Oct 28;114(8):1237-45.

3. Kirmse M, Oertzen-Hagemann V, de Marées M, Bloch W, Platen P. Prolonged collagen peptide supplementation and resistance exercise training

affects body composition in recreationally active men. *Nutrients*. 2019 May 23;11(5):1154.

4.   Jendricke P, Centner C, Zdzieblik D, Gollhofer A, König D. Specific collagen peptides in combination with resistance training improve body composition and regional muscle strength in premenopausal women: A randomized controlled trial. *Nutrients*. 2019 Apr 20;11(4):892.

5.   Zdzieblik D, Jendricke P, Oesser S, Gollhofer A, König D. The influence of specific bioactive collagen peptides on body composition and muscle strength in middle-aged, untrained men: A randomized controlled trial. *Int J Environ Res Public Health*. 2021 Apr 30;18(9):4837.

6.   Yazaki M, Ito Y, Yamada M, et al. Oral ingestion of collagen hydrolysate leads to the transportation of highly concentrated Gly-Pro-Hyp and its hydrolyzed form of Pro-Hyp into the bloodstream and skin. *J Agric Food Chem*. 2017 Mar 22;65(11):2315-22.

7.   Pan L, Ai X, Fu T, et al. In vitro fermentation of hyaluronan by human gut microbiota: Changes in microbiota community and potential degradation mechanism. *Carbohydr Polym*. 2021 Oct 1;269:118313.

8.   Nelson FR, Zvirbulis RA, Zonca et al. The effects of an oral preparation containing hyaluronic acid (Oralvisc®) on obese knee osteoarthritis patients determined by pain, function, bradykinin, leptin, inflammatory cytokines, and heavy water analyses. *Rheumatol Int*. 2015 Jan;35(1):43-52.

9.   Dogné S, Flamion B. Endothelial glycocalyx impairment in disease: Focus on hyaluronan shedding. *Am J Pathol*. 2020 Apr;190(4):768-80.

10. Tan BL, Norhaizan ME. Carotenoids: How effective are they to prevent age-related diseases? *Molecules*. 2019 May 9;24(9):1801.

11. Nakanishi R, Kanazashi M, Tanaka M, et al. Impacts of astaxanthin supplementation on walking capacity by reducing oxidative stress in nursing home residents. *Environ Res Pub Health*. 2022;19:13492.

12. Liu SZ, Ali AS, Campbell MD, et al. Building strength, endurance, and mobility using an astaxanthin formulation with functional training in elderly. *J Cachexia Sarcopenia Muscle*. 2018 Oct;9(5):826-33.

13. Mashhadi NS, Zakerkish M, Mohammadiasl J, Zarei M, Mohammadshahi M, Haghighizadeh MH. Astaxanthin improves glucose metabolism and reduces blood pressure in patients with type 2 diabetes mellitus. *Asia Pac J Clin Nutr*. 2018;27(2):341-46.

14. Mapelli-Brahm P, Barba FJ, Remize F, et al. The impact of fermentation processes on the production, retention and bioavailability of carotenoids: An overview. *Trends in Food Sci Tech*. 2020;99:389-401.

CHAPTER 7

1. Cohen MN, Crane-Kramer GMM, eds. Editors' summation. In *Ancient Health: Skeletal Indicators of Agricultural and Economic Intensification*, University Press of Florida; 2007:320-43.

2. Cordain L. Cereal grains: Humanity's double-edged sword. In Simopoulos AP, ed. *Evolutionary Aspects of Nutrition and Health*. Karger; 1999:19-73.

3. Tito RY, Knights D, Metcalf J, et al. Insights from characterizing extinct human gut microbiomes. *PLoS One.* 2012;7(12):e51146.

4. Adler CJ, Dobney K, Weyrich LS, et al. Sequencing ancient calcified dental plaque shows changes in oral microbiota with dietary shifts of the Neolithic and industrial revolutions. *Nature Genetics.* 2013 Apr;45(4):450-5.

5. Nagar Y, Hershkovitz I. Interrelationship between various aging methods, and their relevance to paleodemography. *Human Evol.* 2004;19: 145-56.

6. Landry MJ, Ward CP, Cunanan KM, et al. Cardiometabolic effects of omnivorous vs. vegan diets in identical twins: A randomized clinical trial. *JAMA Netw Open.* 2023;6(11):e2344457.

7. Berneis KK, Krauss RM. Metabolic origins and clinical significance of LDL heterogeneity. *J Lipid Res.* 2002 Sep;43(9):1363-79.

8. Bali A, Naik R. The impact of a vegan diet on many aspects of health: The overlooked side of veganism. *Cureus.* 2023 Feb 18;15(2):e35148.

9. Fernandez ML. Rethinking dietary cholesterol. *Curr Opin Clin Nutr Metab Care.* 2012 Mar;15(2):117-21.

10. Papandreou C, Moré M, Bellamine A. Trimethylamine N-oxide in relation to cardiometabolic health—cause or effect? *Nutrients.* 2020 May 7;12(5):1330.

11. Kolakowski BM, Miller L, Murray A, Leclair A, Bietlot H, van de Riet JM. Analysis of glyphosate residues in foods from the Canadian retail markets between 2015 and 2017. *J Agric Food Chem.* 2020 May 6;68(18): 5201-11.

12. Chassaing B, Koren O, Goodrich JK, et al. Dietary emulsifiers impact the mouse gut microbiota promoting colitis and metabolic syndrome. *Nature.* 2015 Mar 5;519(7541):92-6.

13. Suez J, Korem T, Zeevi D, et al. Artificial sweeteners induce glucose intolerance by altering the gut microbiota. *Nat. Cell Biol.* 2014;514:181-6.

14. Brantsæter AL, Ydersbond TA, Hoppin JA, Haugen M, Meltzer HM. Organic food in the diet: Exposure and health implications. *Annu Rev Public Health.* 2017 Mar 20;38:295-313.

15. Martin MJ, Thottathil SE, Newman TB. Antibiotics overuse in animal agriculture: A call to action for health care providers. *Am J Public Health*. 2015 Dec;105(12):2409-10.

16. Zioudrou C, Streaty RA, Klee WA. Opioid peptides derived from food proteins: The exorphins. *J Biol Chem*. 1979 Apr 10;254(7):2446-9.

17. Teschemacher H. Opioid receptor ligands derived from food proteins. *Curr Pharm Design*. 2003;9:1331-44.

18. Dohan, FC, Levitt, DR, Kushnir LD. Abnormal behavior after intracerebral injection of polypeptides from wheat gliadin: Possible relevance to schizophrenia. *Pavlovian J Biol Sci*. 1978;13(2):73-82.

19. Casella G, Pozzi R, Cigognetti M, et al. Mood disorders and non-celiac gluten sensitivity. *Minerva Gastroenterol Dietol*. 2017 Mar;63(1):32-7.

20. Cohen MR, Cohen RM, Pickar D, Murphy DL. Naloxone reduces food intake in humans. *Psychosomatic Med*. 1985 Mar/Apr;47(2):1332-8.

21. Drewnowski A, Krahn DD, Demitrack MA, et al. Naloxone, an opiate blocker, reduces the consumption of sweet high-fat foods in obese and lean female binge eaters. *Am J Clin Nutr*. 1995;61:1206-12.

22. Laurens C, Grundler F, Damiot A, et al. Is muscle and protein loss relevant in long-term fasting in healthy men? A prospective trial on physiological adaptations. *J Cachexia Sarcopenia Muscle*. 2021 Dec;12(6):1690-1703.

23. Tinsley GM, Paoli A. Time-restricted eating and age-related muscle loss. *Aging* 2019 Oct 20;11(20):8741-2.

24. Kerem L, Lawson EA. The effects of oxytocin on appetite regulation, food intake and metabolism in humans. *Int J Mol Sci*. 2021 Jul 20;22(14):7737.

25. Martino DJ. The effects of chlorinated drinking water on the assembly of the intestinal microbiome. *Challenges*. 2019 Jan;10(1):10.

CHAPTER 8

1. Holick MF. The vitamin D deficiency pandemic: Approaches for diagnosis, treatment and prevention. *Rev Endocr Metab Disord*. 2017 Jun;18(2):153-65.

2. Nakano T, Chiang KC, Chen CC, et al. Sunlight exposure and phototherapy: Perspectives for healthy aging in an era of COVID-19. *Int J Environ Res Public Health*. 2021 Oct 18;18(20):10950.

3. Rafiq S, Jeppesen PB. Insulin resistance is inversely associated with the status of vitamin D in both diabetic and non-diabetic populations. *Nutrients*. 2021 May 21;13(6):1742.

4. Powner MB, Jeffery G. Light stimulation of mitochondria reduces blood glucose levels. *J Biophotonics*. 2024;17(5):1864.

5.   Cheung IN, Zee PC, Shalman D, et al. Morning and evening blue-enriched light exposure alters metabolic function in normal weight adults. *PLoS One*. 2016 May 18;11(5):e0155601.

6.   Tripkovic L, Lambert H, Hart K, et al. Comparison of vitamin D2 and vitamin D3 supplementation in raising serum 25-hydroxyvitamin D status: A systematic review and meta-analysis. *Am J Clin Nutr*. 2012 Jun;95(6):1357-64.

7.   Mazess RB, Bischoff-Ferrari HA, Dawson-Hughes B. Vitamin D: Bolus is bogus—a narrative review. *JBMR Plus*. 2021 Oct 30;5(12):e10567.

8.   Muñoz A, Grant WB. Vitamin D and cancer: An historical overview of the epidemiology and mechanisms. *Nutrients*. 2022 Mar 30;14(7):1448.

9.   Alfredsson L, Armstrong BK, Butterfield DA, et al. Insufficient sun exposure has become a real public health problem. *Int J Environ Res Public Health*. 2020 Jul 13;17(14):5014.

10. Lotito A, Teramoto M, Cheung M, Becker K, Sukumar D. Serum parathyroid hormone responses to vitamin D supplementation in overweight/obese adults: A systematic review and meta-analysis of randomized clinical trials. *Nutrients*. 2017 Mar 6;9(3):241.

11. Workinger JL, Doyle RP, Bortz J. Challenges in the diagnosis of magnesium status. *Nutrients*. 2018 Sep 1;10(9):1202.

12. Thomas SH, Behr ER. Pharmacological treatment of acquired QT prolongation and torsades de pointes. *Br J Clin Pharmacol*. 2016 Mar;81(3):420-7.

13. Duley L, Gülmezoglu AM, Henderson-Smart DJ, Chou D. Magnesium sulphate and other anticonvulsants for women with pre-eclampsia. *Cochrane Database Syst Rev*. 2010 Nov 10;2010(11):CD000025.

14. Costello RB, Elin RJ, Rosanoff A, et al. Perspective: The case for an evidence-based reference interval for serum magnesium: The time has come. *Adv Nutr*. 2016 Nov 15;7(6):977-93.

15. Razzaque MS. Magnesium: Are we consuming enough? *Nutrients*. 2018 Dec 2;10(12):1863.

16. de Sousa Melo SR, Dos Santos LR, da Cunha Soares T, et al. Participation of magnesium in the secretion and signaling pathways of insulin: An updated review. *Biol Trace Elem Res*. 2022 Aug;200(8):3545-53.

17. Elderawi WA, Naser IA, Taleb MH, Abutair AS. The effects of oral magnesium supplementation on glycemic response among type 2 diabetes patients. *Nutrients*. 2018 Dec 26;11(1):44.

18. Moslehi N, Vafa M, Sarrafzadeh J, Rahimi-Foroushani A. Does magnesium supplementation improve body composition and muscle strength in middle-aged overweight women? A double-blind, placebo-controlled, randomized clinical trial. *Biol Trace Elem Res*. 2013 Jun;153(1-3):111-8.

19. Leung AM, Braverman LE, Pearce EN. History of U.S. iodine fortification and supplementation. *Nutrients*. 2012 Nov 13;4(11):1740-6.

20. Whelton PK, Appel LJ, Sacco RL, et al. Sodium, blood pressure, and cardiovascular disease: Further evidence supporting the American Heart Association sodium reduction recommendations. *Circ*. 2012 Dec 11 126(24):2880-9.

21. Herrick KA, Perrine CG, Aoki Y, Caldwell KL. Iodine status and consumption of key iodine sources in the U.S. population with special attention to reproductive age women. *Nutrients*. 2018 Jul 6;10(7):874.

22. van der Aa MP, Knibbe CA, Boer A, van der Vorst MM. Definition of insulin resistance affects prevalence rate in pediatric patients: A systematic review and call for consensus. *J Pediatr Endocrinol Metab*. 2017 Feb 1;30(2):123-31.

23. Ertuglu LA, Elijovich F, Laffer CL, Kirabo A. Salt-sensitivity of blood pressure and insulin resistance. *Front Physiol*. 2021 Dec 13;12:793924.

24. DiNicolantonio JJ, Niazi AK, Sadaf R, O'Keefe JH, Lucan SC, Lavie CJ. Dietary sodium restriction: Take it with a grain of salt. *Am J Med*. 2013 Nov;126(11):951-5.

25. Messerli FH, Hofstetter L, Syrogiannouli L, et al. Sodium intake, life expectancy, and all-cause mortality. *Eur Heart J*. 2021 Jun 1;42(21): 2103-12.

26. Kodjoe E. Low sodium intake and cardiovascular disease mortality among adults with hypertension. *Int J Cardiol Cardiovasc Risk Prev*. 2022 Dec;15:200158.

27. Dasgupta PK, Liu Y, Dyke JV. Iodine nutrition: Iodine content of iodized salt in the United States. *Environ Sci Technol*. 2008 Feb;42(4):1315-23.

28. Blount BC, Pirkle JL, Osterloh JD, et al. Urinary perchlorate and thyroid hormone levels in adolescent and adult men and women living in the United States. *Environ Health Perspect*. 2006 Dec;154(12)1865-71.

29. Schmutzlerr C, Gotthardt I, Hofmann PJ, et al. Endocrine disruptors and the thyroid gland—a combined *in vitro* and *in vivo* analysis of potential new biomarkers. *Environ Health Perspect*. 2007 Dec;115(Suppl 1):77-83.

30. Welty FK. Omega-3 fatty acids and cognitive function. *Curr Opin Lipidol*. 2023 Feb 1;34(1):12-21.

31. Rehman K, Fatima F, Waheed I, Akash MSH. Prevalence of exposure of heavy metals and their impact on health consequences. *J Cell Biochem*. 2018 Jan;119(1):157-84.

32. Foran SE, Flood JG, Lewandrowski KB. Measurement of mercury levels in concentrated over-the-counter fish oil preparations: Is fish oil healthier than fish? *Arch Pathol Lab Med*. 2003 Dec;127(12):1603-5.

33. Lallès JP. Recent advances in intestinal alkaline phosphatase, inflammation, and nutrition. *Nutr Rev.* 2019 Oct 1;77(10):710-24.

34. Oscarsson J, Hurt-Camejo E. Omega-3 fatty acids eicosapentaenoic acid and docosahexaenoic acid and their mechanisms of action on apolipoprotein B-containing lipoproteins in humans: A review. *Lipids Health Dis.* 2017 Aug 10;16(1):149.

35. Jeromson S, Gallagher IJ, Galloway SD, Hamilton DL. Omega-3 fatty acids and skeletal muscle health. *Mar Drugs.* 2015 Nov 19;13(11):6977-7004.

36. Baker EJ, Miles EA, Burdge GC, Yaqoob P, Calder PC. Metabolism and functional effects of plant-derived omega-3 fatty acids in humans. *Prog Lipid Res.* 2016 Oct;64:30-56.

CHAPTER 9

1.   Gerede A, Nikolettos K, Vavoulidis E, et al. Vaginal microbiome and pregnancy complications: A review. *J Clin Med.* 2024 Jun 30;13(13):3875.

2.   DeGruttola AK, Low D, Mizoguchi A, Mizoguchi E. Current understanding of dysbiosis in disease in human and animal models. *Inflamm Bowel Dis.* 2016 May;22(5):1137-50.

3.   Cani PD, Amar J, Iglesias MA, et al. Metabolic endotoxemia initiates obesity and insulin resistance. *Diabetes.* 1 July 2007; (7): 761-72.

4.   Boutagy NE, McMillan RP, Frisard MI, Hulver MW. Metabolic endotoxemia with obesity: Is it real and is it relevant? *Biochimie.* 2016 May;124:11-20.

5.   Mayorga-Ramos A, Barba-Ostria C, Simancas-Racines D, Guamán LP. Protective role of butyrate in obesity and diabetes: New insights. *Front Nutr.* 2022 Nov 24;9:1067647.

6.   Selle K, Klaenhammer TR. Genomic and phenotypic evidence for probiotic influences of *Lactobacillus gasseri* on human health. *FEMS Microbiol Rev.* 2013 Nov;37(6):915-35.

7.   Coo J, Yu Z, Liu W, et al. Probiotic characteristics of *Bacillus coagulans* and associated implications for human health and diseases, *J Funct Foods.* 2020;64:103643.

8.   Jäger R, Shields KA, Lowery RP, et al. Probiotic *Bacillus coagulans* GBI-30, 6086 reduces exercise-induced muscle damage and increases recovery. *Peer J.* 2016 Jul 21;4:e2276.

9.   Cano R. Unpublished data, 2024.

10. Suez J, Cohen Y, Valdés-Mas R, et al. Personalized microbiome-driven effects of non-nutritive sweeteners on human glucose tolerance. *Cell.* 2022 Sep 1;185(18):3307-28.e19.

11. Shimada S, Tanigawa T, Watanabe T, et al. Involvement of gliadin, a component of wheat gluten, in increased intestinal permeability leading to non-steroidal anti-inflammatory drug-induced small-intestinal damage. *PLoS One*. 2019 Feb 20;14(2):e0211436.

12. Weersma RK, Zhernakova A, Fu J. Interaction between drugs and the gut microbiome. *Gut*. 2020 Aug;69(8):1510-19.

13. Kim J, Yun JM, Kim MK, Kwon O, Cho B. *Lactobacillus gasseri* BNR17 supplementation reduces the visceral fat accumulation and waist circumference in obese adults: A randomized, double-blind, placebo-controlled trial. *J Med Food*. 2018 May;21(5):454-61.

14. Kadooka Y, Sato M, Ogawa A, et al. Effect of *Lactobacillus gasseri* SBT2055 in fermented milk on abdominal adiposity in adults in a randomised controlled trial. *Br J Nutr*. 2013 Nov 14;110(9):1696-703.

15. Wastyk HC, Fragiadakis GK, Perelman D, et al. Gut-microbiota-targeted diets modulate human immune status. *Cell*. 2021 Aug 5;184(16): 4137-53.e14.

16. Abt MC, McKenney PT, Pamer EG. Clostridium difficile colitis: Pathogenesis and host defence. *Nat Rev Microbiol*. 2016 Oct;14(10):609-20.

17. Uebanso T, Shimohata T, Mawatari K, Takahashi A. Functional roles of B-vitamins in the gut and gut microbiome. *Mol Nutr Food Res*. 2020 Sep;64(18):e2000426.

18. Lee JA, Stern JM. Understanding the link between gut microbiome and urinary stone disease. *Curr Urol Rep*. 2019 Mar 22;20(5):19.

19. Méndez-Salazar EO, Martínez-Nava GA. Uric acid extrarenal excretion: The gut microbiome as an evident yet understated factor in gout development. *Rheumatol Int*. 2022 Mar;42(3):403-12.

20. Lasselin J, Lekander M, Benson S, Schedlowski M, Engler H. Sick for science: Experimental endotoxemia as a translational tool to develop and test new therapies for inflammation-associated depression. *Mol Psychiatry*. 2021 Aug;26(8):3672-83.

21. Poutahidis T, Springer A, Levkovich T, et al. Probiotic microbes sustain youthful serum testosterone levels and testicular size in aging mice. *PLoS One*. 2014 Jan 2;9(1):e84877.

22. Knezevic J, Starchl C, Tmava Berisha A, Amrein K. Thyroid-gut-axis: How does the microbiota influence thyroid function? *Nutrients*. 2020 Jun 12;12(6):1769.

23. Chen Y, Singh J, Archer R. Potato starch retrogradation in tuber: Structural changes and gastro-small intestinal digestion in vitro. *Food Hydrocolloids*. 2018;84:552-60.

24. Parnell JA, Reimer RA. Prebiotic fiber modulation of the gut microbiota improves risk factors for obesity and the metabolic syndrome. *Gut Microbes*. 2012 Jan-Feb;3(1):29-34.

Conversion Charts

Conversions are approximate and rounded for practical convenience.

Fermenting and cooking temperatures

Fahrenheit	Celsius
90	30
100	40
120	50
180	80
350	175
375	190

Weight

4 ounces	100g
6 ounces	175g
8 ounces	225g
12 ounces	350g
1 pound	500g
2 pounds	1kg

Volume (liquids)

¼ cup	60ml
½ cup	120ml
¾ cup	180ml
1 cup	240ml
13.5-ounce can	400ml
1 quart	1 litre

Volume (dry ingredients)

Powders e.g flour	1 cup = 125g
Dried legumes e.g lentils	1 cup = 200g
Seeds	1 cup = 150g
Grated cheese	1 cup = 100g

INDEX

abdominal visceral fat
  in body shape, 11–16
  definition of, 10
  gender in, 9
  health implications of, 10–17
  measuring progress with, 76–78, 124
  misinformation about losing, 17,
    19–20 (*see also specific strategies*)
  processed foods in, 32–33
  vs. subcutaneous fat, 10–11
Academy of Nutrition and Dietetics
    (AND), 30–31
ADA. *See* American Diabetes Association
adaptive thermogenesis, 56
addiction, 33, 140–142
additives
  avoiding, 39–40, 137
  in drinking water, 152
  in processed foods, 32, 39, 40
advice. *See* dietary advice
aging
  in body composition and shape, 83–84
  inflammation in, 76
  microbes in, 83–84
  muscle loss as part of, 54, 65–66,
    83–84
agricultural practices, 32, 134, 137–139
Agua de Kefir, 205
AHA. *See* American Heart Association
AIRE device, 104, 107, 190–192
Akkermansia, 194

Alzheimer's disease, 99
American Academy of Pediatrics, 23
American Diabetes Association (ADA), 29
American Heart Association (AHA), 29,
    170, 171
amino acids, 114–115
amoxicillin, 72
amylin, 57
amylopectin A, 36, 139
AND. *See* Academy of Nutrition and
    Dietetics
android (apple-shaped) bodies, 9. *See also*
    abdominal visceral fat
animals
  genetic code of, 8–9, 38
  L. reuteri in, 86, 90
  obesity in, 27
  See also meats
antibiotics
  and *L. reuteri*, 72, 79, 90–91
  and microbiome, 89–91, 182
  natural, 93
  prevalence of prescriptions for, 89
  and SIBO, 100, 187–188
appetite
  fat consumption in, 74
  grains in stimulation of, 36–37,
    139–142, 144
  hormones in, 57, 69, 71
  strategies for reducing, 143–146
  with weight-loss drugs, 51–52

289

ABOUT THE AUTHOR

Dr William Davis is a cardiologist and #1 *New York Times* bestselling author of the *Wheat Belly* series of books, as well as *Undoctored* and *Super Gut*. Recent human clinical trials that Dr. Davis conducted have revealed that it is possible to lose fat weight while preserving muscle, thereby preventing weight regain and enjoying improved body composition, findings that inspired the writing of *SUPER Body*. Dr. Davis is also chief medical officer at Realize Therapeutics Corp., which he cofounded to explore the new science of the microbiome to improve health and appearance, including body composition.

Also by
Dr William Davis

SUPER GUT: A FOUR-WEEK PLAN TO REPROGRAM YOUR
MICROBIOME, RESTORE HEALTH AND LOSE WEIGHT

Trade Paperback ISBN 978-1-399-70181-5

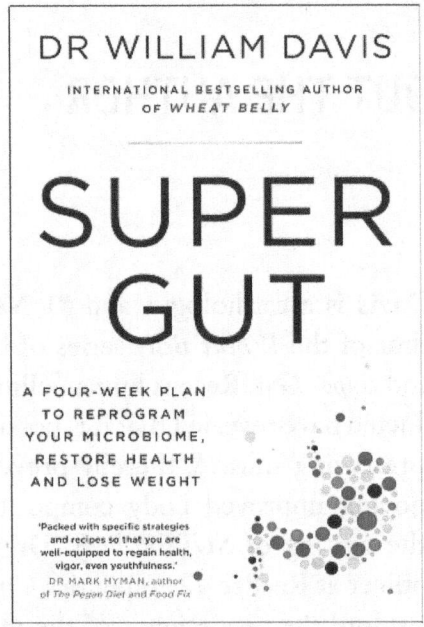

In *Super Gut* Dr William Davis connects the dots between
'gut health' and many common, modern ailments and complaints.
1 in 3 people have SIBO (small intestinal bacterial overgrowth),
which causes a long list of health issues and illnesses; it is a silent and
profound epidemic created by the absence of microbial species that
our ancestors had even 50–100 years ago, which have been erased by
the industrialisation of food and medicine.

Super Gut shares a four-week plan to reprogram your microbiome,
getting to the root of many diseases, improving levels of oxytocin and
overall brain health, and promoting anti-aging and weight loss.
Dr William Davis provides not just the science and case studies
but also more than 40 recipes and solutions. He ensures readers
understand the science, diagnose their gut issues, eradicate them and
maintain their long-term health.